DR. ACKERMAN'S BOOK OF WEST HIGHLAND WHITE TERRIERS

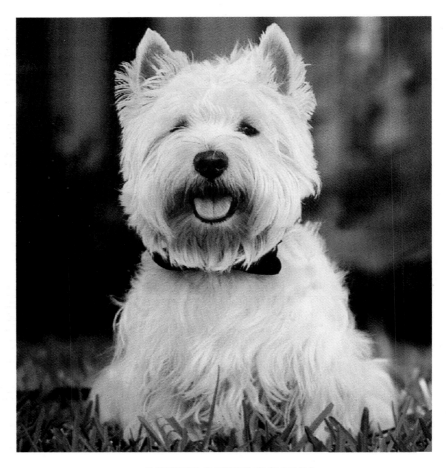

LOWELL ACKERMAN DVM

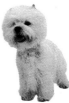

BB-110

Overleaf: West Highland White Terrier
photographed by Gillian Lisle.

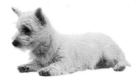

The author has exerted every effort to ensure that medical information mentioned in this book is in accord with current recommendations and practice at the time of publication. However, in view of the ongoing advances in veterinary medicine, the reader is urged to consult with his veterinarian regarding individual health issues.

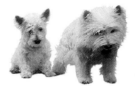

Photographers: Judy Arenz, Wil de Veer, Isabelle Francais, Daphne Gentry, Jeff Greene, Judith Iby, Gillian Lisle, Ron Reagan, Vincent Serbin.

The presentation of pet products in this book is strictly for instructive purposes only; it does not necessarily constitute an endorsement by the author, publisher, owner of dogs portrayed, or any other contributors.

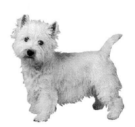

© 1997 by LOWELL ACKERMAN DVM

Distributed in the UNITED STATES to the Pet Trade by T.F.H. Publications, Inc., One T.F.H. Plaza, Neptune City, NJ 07753; distributed in the UNITED STATES to the Bookstore and Library Trade by National Book Network, Inc. 4720 Boston Way, Lanham MD 20706; in CANADA to the Pet Trade by H & L Pet Supplies Inc., 27 Kingston Crescent, Kitchener, Ontario N2B 2T6; Rolf C. Hagen Inc., 3225 Sartelon St. Laurent-Montreal Quebec H4R 1E8; in CANADA to the Book Trade by Vanwell Publishing Ltd., 1 Northrup Crescent, St. Catharines, Ontario L2M 6P5 ; in ENGLAND by T.F.H. Publications, PO Box 15, Waterlooville PO7 6BQ; in AUSTRALIA AND THE SOUTH PACIFIC by T.F.H. (Australia), Pty. Ltd., Box 149, Brookvale 2100 N.S.W., Australia; in NEW ZEALAND by Brooklands Aquarium Ltd. 5 McGiven Drive, New Plymouth, RD1 New Zealand; in Japan by T.F.H. Publications, Japan—Jiro Tsuda, 10-12-3 Ohjidai, Sakura, Chiba 285, Japan; in SOUTH AFRICA by Lopis (Pty) Ltd., P.O. Box 39127, Booysens, 2016, Johannesburg, South Africa. Published by T.F.H. Publications, Inc.
MANUFACTURED IN THE
UNITED STATES OF AMERICA
BY T.F.H. PUBLICATIONS, INC.

CONTENTS

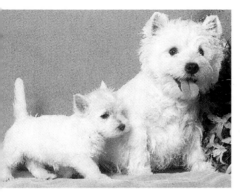

DEDICATION · 4
PREFACE · 4
BIOGRAPHY · 5
BREED HISTORY by Daphne Gentry · 6
MIND & BODY · 10
Conformation & Physical Characteristics ·
Coat Color, Care,& Condition · Behavior &
Personality of the Active West Highland White
Terrier
SELECTING · 16
Sources · Medical Screening · Behavioral
Screening · Organizations You Should
Know About

FEEDING AND NUTRITION · 28
Commercial Dog Foods · Puppy
Requirements · Adult Diets
· Geriatric Diets · Medical Condi-
tions and Diet
HEALTH · 36
Two to Three Weeks of Age · Six
toTwenty
Weeks of Age
· Four to Twelve Months of Age · One to Seven Years of Age
·Senior West Highland White Terriers
MEDICAL PROBLEMS · 48
Cataracts · Craniomandibular Osteopathy · Elbow Dysplasia
· Epidermal Dysplasia · Glaucoma ·
Globoid Cell Leukodystrophy · Hip
Dysplasia · Hypothyroidism · Inhalant
Allergies · Legg-Calve-Perthes Disease ·
Liver Disease Due to Copper Accumulation · Medial Patellar
Luxation · Pulmonic Stenosis · Von Willebrand's Disease
INFECTIONS & INFESTATIONS · 66
Fleas · Ticks · Mange · Heartworm · Intestinal Parasites
· Viral Infections · Canine Cough
FIRST AID by Judy Iby, RVT · 78
Temperature · Capillary Refill Time
and Gum Color · Heart Rate, Pulse,
and Respirations · Preparing for an Emergency ·
Emergency Muzzle · Antifreeze Poisoning · Bee Stings ·
Bleeding · Bloat · Burns · Cardiopulmonary Resuscita-
tion (CPR) · Chocolate Toxicosis · Choking · Dog Bites ·
Drowning · Electrocution · Eyes · Fish Hooks · Foreign
Objects · Heatstroke · Poisons · Porcupine Quills ·
Seizure (Convulsion or Fit) · Severe Trauma · Shock
·Skunks · Snake Bites · Toad Poisoning · Vaccination
Reaction
RECOMMENDED READING · 95

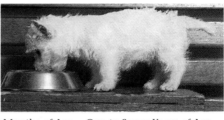
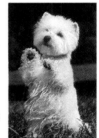
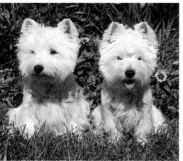

DEDICATION

To my wonderful wife Susan and my three adorable children, Nadia, Rebecca, and David.

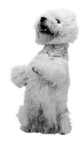

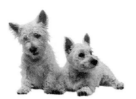

PREFACE

Keeping your West Highland White Terrier healthy is the most important job that you, as owner, can do. Whereas there are many books available that deal with breed qualities, conformation, and show characteristics, this may be the only book available dedicated entirely to the preventative health care of the West Highland White Terrier. This information has been compiled from a variety of sources and assembled here to provide you with the most up-to-date advice available.

This book will take you through the important stages of selecting your pet, screening it for inherited medical and behavioral problems, meeting its nutritional needs, and seeing that it receives optimal medical care.

So, enjoy the book and use the information to keep your West Highland White Terrier the healthiest it can be for a long, full and rich life.

Lowell Ackerman DVM

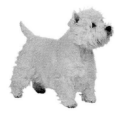

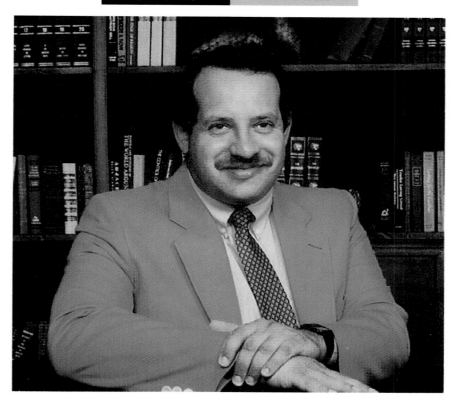

BIOGRAPHY

D
r. Lowell Ackerman is a world-renowned veterinary clinician, author, lecturer and radio personality. He is a Diplomate of the American College of Veterinary Dermatology and is a consultant in the fields of dermatology, nutrition and genetics. Dr. Ackerman is the author of 34 books and over 150 book chapters and articles. He also hosts a national radio show on pet health care and moderates a site on the World Wide Web dedicated to pet health care issues (http://www.familyinternet.com/pet/pet-vet.htm).

BREED HISTORY

by Daphne Gentry

**THE GENESIS OF THE MODERN
WEST HIGHLAND WHITE TERRIER**

The West Highland White Terrier, affectionately known as the Westie, is a "small, game, well-balanced hardy looking terrier" native to the Scottish Highlands. There, where jagged and bare rocks stand out on hillsides concealing fox and badger, was the perfect climate for the development of a dog able to go to ground and drive vermin

Facing page: Of all the terrier breeds, there is none more friendly and loyal than the adorable West Highland White Terrier.

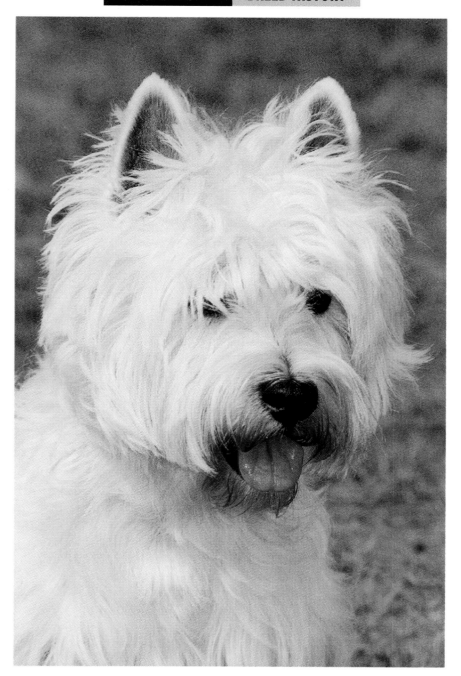

into the open. Such a dog needed to be relatively small yet robust; to have a thick wiry and almost waterproof coat; short, strong legs and feet; powerful jaws; and, most importantly, no small amount of courage. Such is the description of that dog we today know as the West Highland White Terrier.

While the origins of some breeds are easily traced, that of the Westie is not. There are, of course, many and varying claims ranging from the Westie descending from those legendary Spanish white terriers that were kept aboard ship to kill rats who swam ashore following the defeat of the Spanish Armada in 1588, to being simply the white variation of the Cairn or Scottish Terriers. Those who follow the storyline that the Westie descends from those dogs surviving the Armada defeat claim that the "terrieres or earthe dogges" James I (1566-1625) requested be sent to a friend in France from Argyll were in truth the forerunners of the Westie. Truthfully, however, the origins of the breed are cloaked in the clouds that hang over the highlands from which he came.

While it is unlikely that the actual origin of the Westie will ever be determined, the breed was on its way to being well-

defined by the mid-Victorian period. In the final decade of the nineteenth century, a Captain Mackie described the Poltalloch dogs, those which would soon be called Westies, as being of a "linty white" color, "cream in an otherwise white dog and the skin of the body is generally pigmented." The same writer noted a "dorsal line of cream or fawn" in the dogs he saw.

The breed found its way across the Atlantic early in the twentieth century, even before it had been recognized under the current name in England. The individual who imported the first Westie may, like the origins of the breed itself, be cloaked in anonymity but certainly a case can be made for that person to be Mrs. H. M. Harriman, although Mrs. Robert Low Bacon and Robert Geolet each laid claims to have been the first to import a Westie to the United States.

The American Kennel Club accepted the first registrations for its stud book in 1908 under the Roseneath Terrier designation. Within a year, however, the breed's name in both the stud book and the show catalogs was the West Highland White Terrier; the first actually to be registered under that breed designation was the bitch Sky Lady, who along with her son and another bitch were imported by R. D. Humphrey and Philip Boyer. The first Westie to be registered in Canada was named Calehaig and had been whelped in Scotland; he was brought to Canada the year following his 1908 birth. It was another three years before shows including classes for the breed were held in Canada.

Through the years the Westie has enjoyed success in all elements of dog events. Today the West Highland White Terrier can be found in the show ring and the obedience ring, in the earths of den trials and the track of the field; he is also to be found in nursing homes in the role of therapy dog; he is to be found as companion to families of one or ten; but wherever he is found, he exhibits that "no small amount of self esteem" which sets him apart and endears him to all those who know him.

Westies are a hardy breed whose small size allows them to chase burrowing animals through confined spaces. This Westie's hunting instincts still exist today as he chases his ball through a narrow tube.

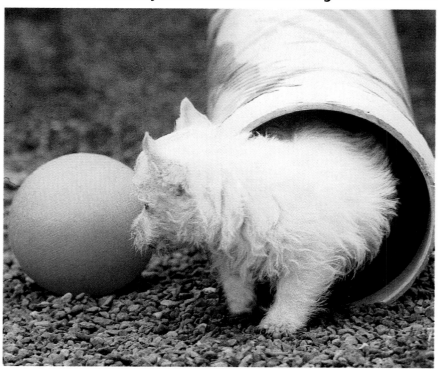

MIND & BODY

**PHYSICAL AND BEHAVIORAL TRAITS OF THE
WEST HIGHLAND WHITE TERRIER**

The small, snow-white Westie is a favorite of children and adults. Who can resist this little fellow's impish charm and good looks? But the West Highland White Terrier is more than the placid pet he may appear to be. This is an energetic, opinionated dog bred to pursue rats and other vermin. He has personality plus.

Facing page: The West Highland White Terrier is a small, game, energetic dog with plenty of personality and no lack of self-esteem.

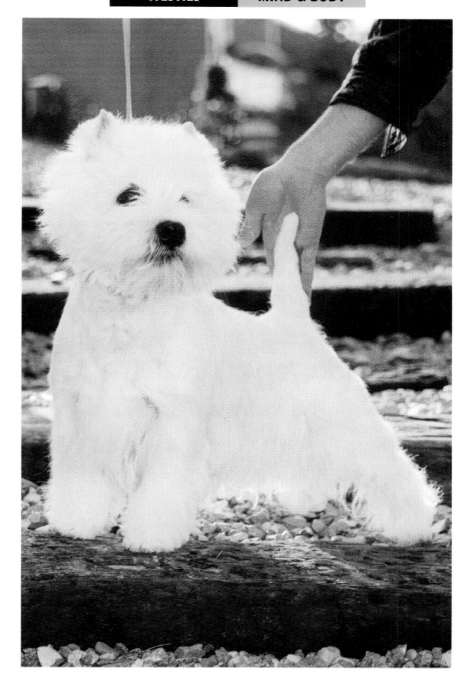

CONFORMATION AND PHYSICAL CHARACTERISTICS

This is not a book about show dogs, so information here will not deal with the conformation of champions and how to select one. The purpose of this chapter is to provide basic information about the stature of a West Highland White Terrier and qualities of a physical nature.

Clearly, beauty is in the eye of the beholder. And, since standards come and standards go, measuring your dog against some imaginary yardstick does little for you or your dog. Just because your dog isn't a show champion, doesn't mean that he or she is any less of a family member. And, just because a dog is a champion doesn't mean that he or she is not a genetic time bomb waiting to go off.

When breeders and those interested in showing West Highland White Terriers are selecting dogs, they are looking for those qualities that match the breed "standard." This standard, however, is of an imaginary West Highland White Terrier and it changes from time to time and from country to country. Thus, the conformation and physical characteristics that pet owners should concentrate on are somewhat different and much more practical.

The breed standard for the

Today's Westies still possess the strong field capabilities of their ancestors.

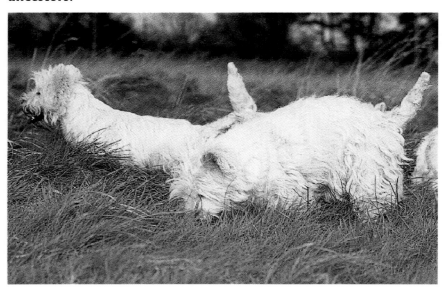

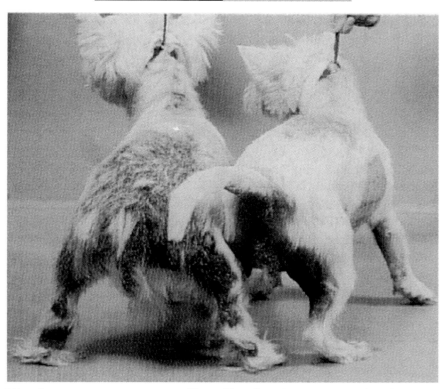

Westies are more prone to flea allergies than some other breeds. These two unrelated Westies are badly affected.

West Highland White Terrier calls for a small, game, well-balanced, hardy looking terrier, exhibiting good showmanship, possessed with no small amount of self-esteem, strongly built, deep in chest and back ribs with a straight back and powerful hindquarters on muscular legs, and exhibiting in marked degree a great combination of strength and activity. The ideal size is eleven inches at the withers for dogs and ten inches for bitches.

COAT COLOR, CARE AND CONDITION

The West Highland White Terrier should be, by definition, white and there will be black pigmentation associated with the nose, lips, eye-rims, foot pads, nails and the hue of the skin. The eyes are generally dark in color and most breeders find that light-colored eyes are undesirable, although there are no health reasons for this preference.

Westies have a double coat in which the outer guard hairs are straight and hard. The coat tends to be shorter on the neck and shoulders. The undercoat is soft and dense. Breeders of show dogs spend an inordinate amount of time grooming the Westie for a certain look. The pet Westie is much easier to maintain, yet still requires regular brushing and visits to the groomers. Clipping tends to soften the coat while breeders tend to "pluck" and "strip" to maintain the harsh, wiry outer coat.

The West Highland White Terrier is prone to several different skin problems and they can affect the appearance. Allergies are extremely common in the breed and result in licking and scratching, especially involving the feet, face, armpits and groin. The skin becomes red and eventually black; hair loss is often evident as well and the skin may become thickened and cracked. Epidermal hyperplasia in a congenital skin problem that typically is seen first in dogs less than 6 months of age. It is often complicated by yeast infection. It can look very similar to allergies and the two are not always easy to differentiate.

The incidence of skin problems is mentioned here because many Westies eventually require medicated shampoos. Suitable ingredients for mild cases include selenium disulfide, sulfur and salicylic acid. Tar shampoos may stain the coat and benzoyl peroxides tend to irritate the skin and dry it out further.

BEHAVIOR AND PERSONALITY OF THE ACTIVE WEST HIGHLAND WHITE TERRIER

Behavior and personality are two qualities which are hard to standardize within a breed. The breed standards for the West Highland White Terrier calls for it to be possessed with no small amount of self-esteem, alert, gay, courageous and self-reliant, but friendly. These are all valued traits in any breed. Although generalizations are difficult to make, most West Highland White Terriers are very alert and people-oriented. In fact, they have been referred to as "people-pleasing" dogs. They are happy to play, work or just keep you company. Whether they are shy or vicious has something to do with their genetics, but also is determined by the socialization and training they receive.

Behavior and personality are incredibly important in dogs and there seems to be quite evident extremes in the West Highland White Terrier. The ideal West

Highland White Terrier is neither aggressive nor neurotic but rather a loving family member with good self-esteem and acceptance of position in the family "pack." Because the West Highland White Terrier is a willful dog and can cause much damage, it is worth spending the time when selecting a pup to pay attention to any evidence of personality problems. It is also imperative that *all* West Highland White Terriers be obedience trained. Like any dog, they have the potential to be unruly without appropriate training; consider obedience classes mandatory for your sake and that of your dog.

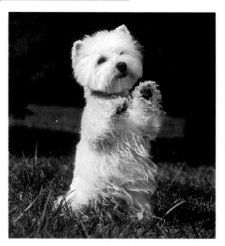

Westies are affectionate, fun-loving dogs who are known as "people-pleasers." This little guy will do anything for his owner's attention.

Although many Westies are happy to sleep the day away in bed or on a sofa, most enjoy having a purpose in their day and that makes them excellent working dogs. They do not need long daily walks but they do appreciate events that involve family members. All West Highland White Terriers should attend obedience classes and they need to learn limits to unacceptable behaviors. A well-loved and well-controlled West Highland White Terrier is certain to be a valued family member.

For pet owners, there are several activities to which your West Highland White Terrier is well-suited. They not only make great walking and jogging partners but they are also excellent community volunteers. The breed seems ideally suited to standing still for kisses, hugs and petting that can last for hours at a time. The loyal and loving West Highland White Terrier will also be your personal guard dog if properly trained; aggressiveness and viciousness do not fit into the equation.

For West Highland White Terrier enthusiasts who want to get into more competitive aspects of the dog world, showing, hunting, obedience, tracking and den trials are all activities that can be considered.

SELECTING

**WHAT YOU NEED TO KNOW TO FIND THE BEST
WEST HIGHLAND WHITE TERRIER PUPPY**

Owning the perfect West Highland White Terrier rarely happens by accident. On the other hand, owning a genetic dud is almost always the result of an impulse purchase and failure to do even basic research.

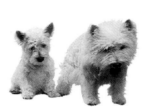

Buying this book is a major step in understanding the situation and making intelligent choices.

Facing page: Although West Highland White Terrier puppies are adorable and irresistible, the decision to own one should be made with careful consideration.

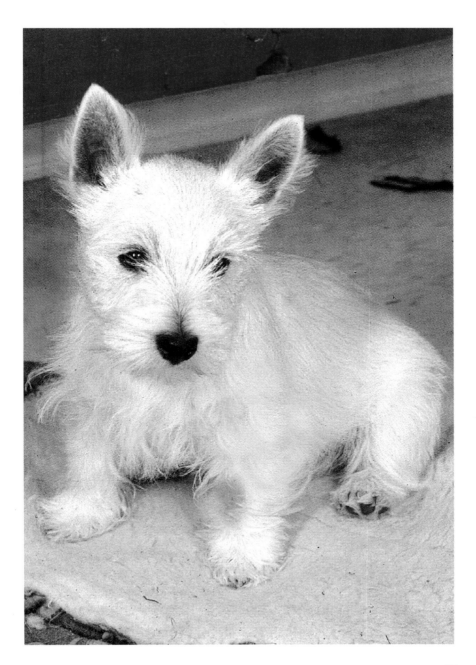

SOURCES

Recently, a large survey was done to determine whether there were more problems seen in animals adopted from pet stores, breeders, private owners or animal shelters. Somewhat surprisingly, there didn't appear to be any major difference in total number of problems seen from these sources. What was different were the kinds of problems seen in each source. Thus, you can't rely on any one source because there are no standards by which judgments can be made. Most veterinarians will recommend that you select a "good breeder" but there is no way to identify such an individual. A breeder of champion show dogs may also be a breeder of genetic defects.

The best approach is to select a pup from a source that regularly performs genetic screening and has documentation to prove it. If you are intending to be a pet owner, don't worry about whether your pup is show quality. A mark here or there that might disqualify the pup as a show winner has absolutely no impact on its ability to be a lov-

When selecting your Westie pup, check that his parents have been genetically screened and have proper documentation.

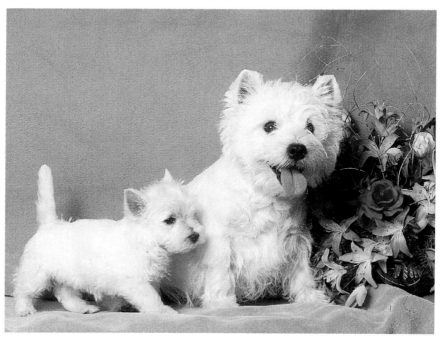

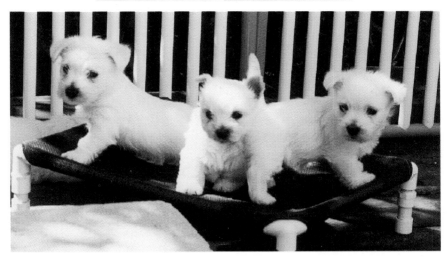

As soon as you take your pick of the litter, have your veterinarian check your Westie for medical and behavioral problems.

ing and healthy pet. Also, the vast majority of dogs will be neutered and not used for breeding anyway. Concentrate on the things that are important.

MEDICAL SCREENING

Whether you are dealing with a breeder, a breed rescue group, a shelter or a pet store, your approach should be the same. You want to identify a West Highland White Terrier that you can live with and screen it for medical and behavioral problems before you make it a permanent family member. If the source you select has not done the important testing needed, make sure they will offer you a health/temperament guarantee before you remove the dog from the premises to have the work done yourself. If this is not acceptable, or they are offering an exchange-only policy, keep moving; this isn't the right place for you to get a dog. As soon as you purchase a Westie, pup or adult, go to your veterinarian for thorough evaluation and testing.

Pedigree analysis is best left to true enthusiasts but there are some things that you can do, even as a novice. Inbreeding is to be discouraged so check out your four- or five-generation pedigree and look for names that appear repeatedly. Reputable breeders will usually not allow inbreeding at least three generations back in the puppy's pedigree. Also ask the breeder to provide OFA and CERF registration numbers on all ancestors in the pedigree for which testing is done. If there are a lot of gaps, the breeder has some explaining to do.

The screening procedure is easier if you select an older dog. Animals can be registered for hips and elbows as young as two years of age by the Orthopedic Foundation for Animals and by one year of age by Genetic Disease Control. This is your insurance against hip dysplasia and elbow dysplasia later in life. Although West Highland White Terriers now have a relatively low incidence of these orthopedic problems, it is because of the efforts of conscientious breeders who have been doing the appropriate testing. A verbal testimonial that they've never heard of the condition in their lines is not adequate and probably means they really don't know if they have a problem. Move along.

Evaluation is somewhat more complicated in the West Highland White Terrier puppy. The PennHip™ procedure can determine risk for developing hip dysplasia in pups as young as 16 weeks of age. For pups younger

This Westie is showing off his fine form. Groomed for the ring, no terrier can compare to the champion Westie.

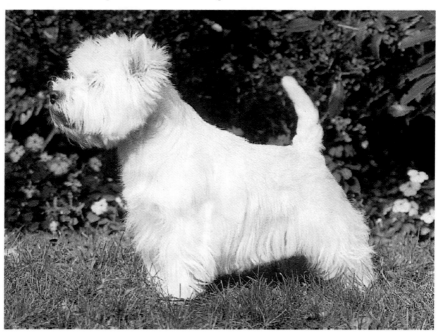

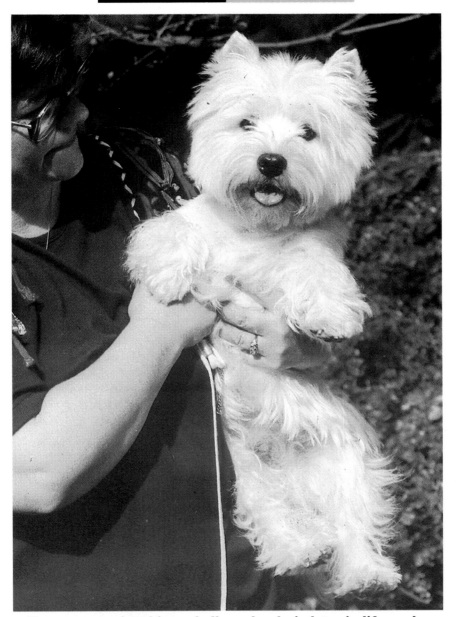

To ensure against hip and elbow dysplasia later in life, make sure the dog you choose is registered with the Orthopedic Foundation for Animals and by Genetic Disease Control.

than that, you should request copies of OFA or GDC registration for both parents. If the parents haven't both been registered, their hip and elbow status should be considered unknown and questionable.

All West Highland White Terriers, regardless of age, should be screened for evidence of von Willebrand's disease. This can be accomplished with a simple blood test. The incidence is high enough in the breed that there is no excuse for not performing the test. For animals older than one year of age, your veterinarian will also want to take a

If your veterinarian suspects a problem, she may need to draw some blood from your Westie.

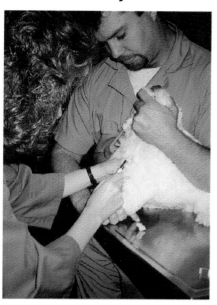

heartworm test, urinalysis and evaluation of feces for internal parasites.

Your veterinarian should also perform a very thorough ophthalmologic (eye) examination. The most common eye problems in West Highland White Terriers are cataracts, persistent pupillary membranes and retinal dysplasia. It is best to acquire a pup whose parents have both been screened for heritable eye diseases and certified "clear" by organizations such as CERF (see below). If this has been the case, an examination by your veterinarian is probably sufficient and referral to an ophthalmologist is only necessary if recommended by your veterinarian.

BEHAVIORAL SCREENING

Medical screening is important but don't forget temperament. More dogs are killed each year for behavioral reasons than for all medical problems combined. Temperament testing is a valuable although not infallible tool in the screening process. The reason that temperament is so important is that many dogs are eventually destroyed because they exhibit undesirable behaviors. Although not all behaviors are evident in young pups (e.g. aggression often takes many

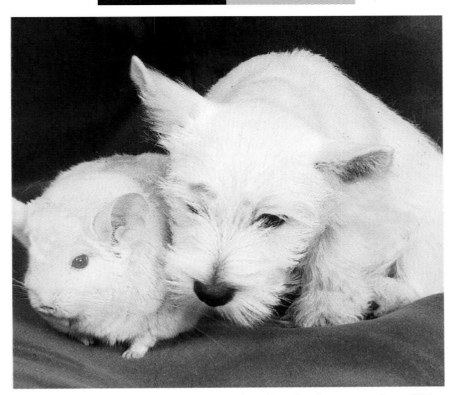

If you properly socialize your Westie when he is young, he will be able to make friends with just about anybody—or anything!

months to manifest itself), detecting anxious and fearful pups (and avoiding them) can be very important in the selection process. Traits most identifiable in the young pup include: fear; excitability; low pain threshold; extreme submission; and noise sensitivity.

There are many different techniques available and a complete discussion is beyond the scope of this book. I encourage you to investigate further.

Pups can be evaluated for temperament as early as seven to eight weeks of age. Some behaviorists, breeders and trainers recommend objective testing where scores are given in several different categories. Others are more casual about the process since it only a crude indicator anyway. In general, the evaluation takes place in three stages, by someone the pup has not been exposed to. The testing is not done within 72 hours of vaccination or surgery. First, the pup is observed and handled to determine its sociability. Puppies with obvious undesirable traits such as shyness, overactivity or uncontrollable biting may turn out to be unsuitable. Second, the desired pup is separated from the others and then observed for how they respond when played with and called. Third, the pup should be stimulated in various ways and their responses noted. Suitable activities include lying the pup on its side, grooming it, clipping its nails, gently grasping it around the muzzle and testing its reactions to noise. In a study conducted at the Psychology Department of Colorado State University, the staff also found that heart rate was a good indicator in this third stage of evaluation. Actually, they noted the resting heart rate, stimulated the pups with a loud noise and measured how long it took the heart rate to recover to resting levels. Most pups recovered within 36 seconds. Dogs that took considerably longer were more likely to be anxious.

Puppy aptitude tests (PAT) can be given in which a numerical score is given for eleven dif-

Make sure your dog has been screened for any signs of heritable eye diseases and certified "clear" by the Canine Eye Registration Foundation. Dogs that fail the eye exam should not be bred.

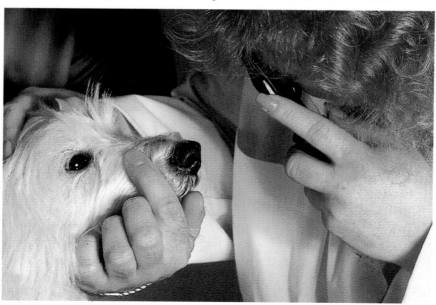

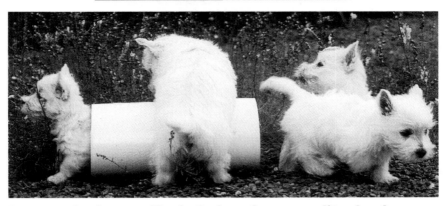

Puppy aptitude tests effectively show the personality of each puppy, revealing which puppies would best suit which potential owners.

ferent traits, with a "1" representing the most assertive or aggressive expression of a trait and a "6" representing disinterest, independence or inaction. The traits assessed in the PAT include: social attraction to people, following, restraint, social dominance, elevation (lifting off ground by evaluator), retrieve, touch sensitivity, sound sensitivity, prey/chase drive, stability, and energy level. Although the tests do not absolutely predict behaviors, they do tend to do well at predicting puppies at behavioral extremes.

ORGANIZATIONS YOU SHOULD KNOW ABOUT

Project TEACH™ (Training and Education in Animal Care and Health) is a voluntary accreditation process for those individuals selling animals to the public. It is administered by Pet Health Initiative, Inc. (PHI) and provides instruction on genetic screening as well as many other aspects of proper pet care. TEACH-accredited sources screen animals for a variety of medical, behavioral and infectious diseases *before* they are sold. Project TEACH™ supports the efforts of registries such as OFA, GDC and CERF and recommends that all animals sold be registered with the appropriate agencies. For more information on Project TEACH™, send a self-addressed stamped envelope to Pet Health Initiative, P.O. Box 12093, Scottsdale, AZ 85267-2093.

The Orthopedic Foundation for Animals (OFA) is a nonprofit organization established in 1966 to collect and disseminate information concerning orthopedic diseases of animals and to establish control programs to lower the incidence of orthopedic diseases in animals. A registry is maintained for both hip dysplasia and elbow dysplasia. The ultimate purpose of OFA certification is to provide information to dog owners to assist in the selection of good breeding animals; therefore, attempts to get a dysplastic dog certified will only hurt the breed by perpetuation of the disease. For more information contact your veterinarian or the Orthopedic Foundation for Animals, 2300 Nifong Blvd., Columbia, MO 65201.

The Institute for Genetic Disease Control in Animals (GDC) is a nonprofit organization founded in 1990 and maintains an open registry for orthopedic problems but does not compete with OFA. In an open registry like GDC, owners, breeders, veterinarians, and scientists can trace the genetic history of any particular dog once that dog and close relatives have been registered. At the present time, the GDC operates open registries for hip dysplasia, elbow dysplasia, and osteochondrosis. The GDC is currently developing guidelines for registries of Legg-Calve-

These Westie puppies are ready to take on the world! However, do not let your puppy outside unless he is fully vaccinated and under supervision.

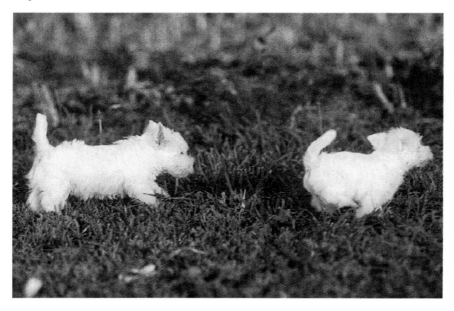

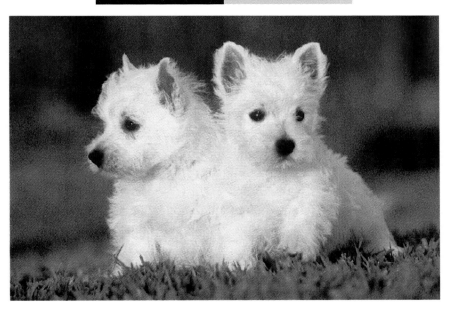

Give your Westie puppies the best possible start in life by making sure their parents have been screened free of all heritable diseases and by providing them with the best possible medical care.

Perthes disease, craniomandibular osteopathy, and medial patellar luxation. All are significant in the West Highland White Terrier. For more information, contact the Institute for Genetic Disease Control in Animals, P.O. Box 222, Davis, CA 95617.

The Canine Eye Registration Foundation (CERF) is an international organization devoted to eliminating hereditary eye diseases from purebred dogs. This organization is similar to OFA that helps eliminate disease like hip dysplasia. CERF is a non-profit organization that screens and certifies purebreds as free of heritable eye diseases. Dogs are evaluated by veterinary eye specialists and finding are then submitted to CERF for documentation.

The goal is to identify purebreds without heritable eye problems so they can be used for breeding. Dogs being considered for breeding programs should be screened and certified by CERF on an annual basis since not all problems are evident in puppies. For more information on CERF, write to CERF, SCC-A, Purdue University, West Lafayette, IN 47907.

FEEDING & NUTRITION

WHAT YOU MUST CONSIDER EVERY DAY TO FEED YOUR WEST HIGHLAND WHITE TERRIER THROUGH HIS LIFETIME

N utrition is one of the most important aspects of raising a healthy West Highland White Terrier and yet it is often the source of much controversy between breeders, veterinarians, pet owners and dog food manufacturers. However, most of these arguments have more to do with

Facing page: Your Westie may want to choose his own snacks, but make sure you, as his owner, choose a nutritional and balanced diet for your pet. This is Bailey's Irish Creme of Acoma owned by Kathleen Spradleg.

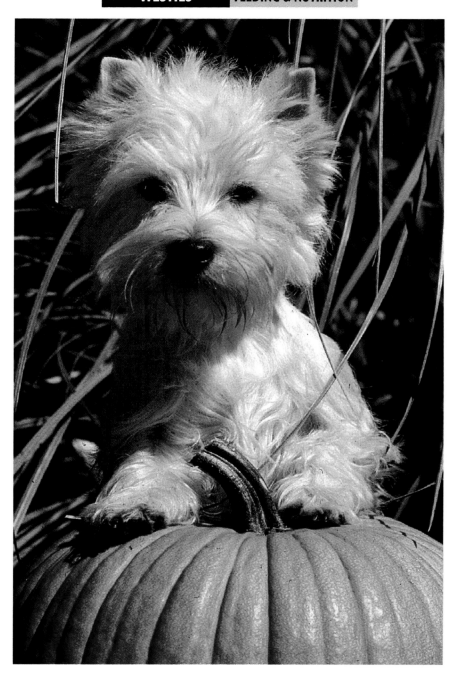

marketing than with science. Let's first take a look at dog foods and then determine the needs of our dog. This chapter will concentrate of feeding the pet West Highland White Terrier rather than breeding or working animals.

COMMERCIAL DOG FOODS

Most dog foods are sold based on marketing (i.e., how to make a product appealing to owners while meeting the needs of dogs). Some foods are marketed on the basis of their protein

Ideally, you want to choose a diet for your Westie that meets his nutritional needs and is appropriate for his stage of life.

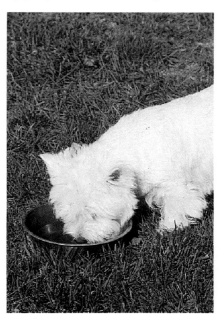

content; others based on a "special" ingredient and some are sold because they don't contain certain ingredients (e.g., preservatives, soy). We want a dog food that specifically meets our dog's needs, is economical and causes few if any problems. Most foods come in dry, semi-moist and canned forms. Some can now be purchased frozen. The "dry" foods are the most economical, contain the least fat and the most preservatives. The canned foods are the most expensive (they're 75% water), usually contain the most fat, and have the least preservatives. Semi-moist foods are expensive, high in sugar content and I do not recommend them for any dogs.

When you're selecting a commercial diet, make sure the food has been assessed by feeding trials for a specific life stage, not just by nutrient analysis. This statement is usually located not far from the ingredient label. In the United States, these trials are performed in accordance with American Association of Feed Control Officials (AAFCO) and, in Canada, by the Canadian Veterinary Medical Association. This certification is important because it has been found that dog foods currently on the market that provide only

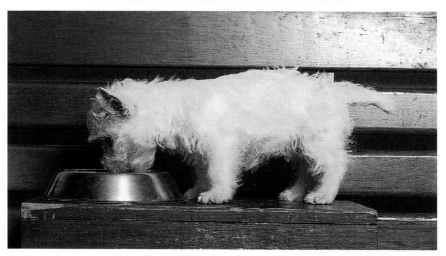

By two months of age, puppies should be fed puppy food and be put on a "growth" diet until they are nine to twelve months.

chemical analyses and calculated values but no feeding trial may not provide adequate nutrition. The feeding trials show that the diets meet minimal, not optimal standards. However, they are the best tests we currently have.

PUPPY REQUIREMENTS

Soon after pups are born, and certainly within the first 24 hours, they should begin nursing their mother. This provides them with colostrum which is an antibody-rich milk that helps protect them from infection for their first few months of life. Pups should be allowed to nurse for at least six weeks before they are completely weaned from their mother. Supplemental feeding may be started by as early as three weeks of age.

By two months of age, pups should be fed puppy food. They are now in an important growth phase. Nutritional deficiencies and/or imbalances during this time of life are more devastating that at any other time. Also, this is not the time to overfeed pups or provide them with "performance" rations.

Pups should be fed "growth" diets until they are 9-12 months of age. Pups will initially need to be fed two to three meals daily until they are 12 months old, then once to twice daily (preferably twice) when they are converted to adult food. Proper growth diets should be selected based on acceptable feeding trials designed for growing pups. If you can't tell by reading the label, ask your veterinarian for feeding advice.

Remember that pups need "balance" in their diets and avoid the temptation to supplement with protein, vitamins, or minerals. Calcium supplements have been implicated as a cause of bone and cartilage deformity, especially in large breed puppies. Puppy diets are already heavily fortified with calcium, and supplements tend to unbalance the mineral intake. There is more than adequate proof that these supplements are responsible for many bone deformities seen in these growing dogs.

ADULT DIETS

The goal of feeding adult dogs is one of "maintenance." They have already done the growing they are going to do and are unlikely to have the digestive problems of elderly dogs. In general, dogs can do well on maintenance rations containing predominantly plant or animal-based ingredients as long as that ration has been specifically formulated to meet maintenance level requirements. This contention should be supported by studies performed by the manufacturer in accordance with AAFCO (American Association of Feed Control Officials). In Canada, these products should be certified by the Canadian Veterinary Medical Association to meet maintenance requirements.

There's nothing wrong with feeding a cereal-based diet to dogs on maintenance rations and they are the most economical. When comparing maintenance rations, it must be appreciated that these diets must meet the "minimum" requirements for confined dogs, not necessarily optimal levels. Most dogs will benefit when fed diets that contain easily digested ingredients that provide nutrients at least slightly above minimum requirements. Typically, these foods will be intermediate in price between the most expensive super-premium diets and the cheapest generic diets. Select only those diets that have been substantiated by feeding trials to meet maintenance requirements, those that contain wholesome ingredients, and those recommended by your veterinarian. Don't select based on price alone, on company advertising, or on total protein content.

GERIATRIC DIETS

West Highland White Terriers are considered elderly when they are about seven years of age and there are certain changes

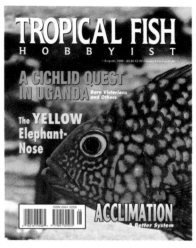

Since 1952, Tropical Fish Hobbyist has been the source of accurate, up-to-the-minute, and fascinating information on every facet of the aquarium hobby. Join the more than 60,000 devoted readers worldwide who wouldn't miss a single issue.

Subscribe right now so you don't miss a single copy!

SM 402

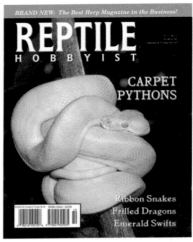

that occur as dogs age that alter their nutritional requirements. As pets age, their metabolism slows and this must be accounted for. If maintenance rations are fed in the same amounts while metabolism is slowing, weight gain may result. Obesity is the last thing one wants to contend with in an elderly pet, since it increases their risk of several other health-related problems. As pets age, most of their organs function not as well as in youth. The digestive system, the liver, pancreas and gallbladder are not functioning at peak effect. The intestines have more difficulty extracting all the nutrients from the food consumed. A gradual decline in kidney function is considered a normal part of aging.

A responsible approach to geriatric nutrition is to realize that degenerative changes are a normal part of aging. Our goal is to minimize the potential damage done by taking this into account while the dog is still well. If we wait until an elderly dog is ill before we change the diet, we have a much harder job.

Elderly dogs need to be treated as individuals. While some benefit from the nutrition found in "senior" diets, others might do better on the highly digestible puppy and super-premium diets. These latter diets provide an excellent blend of digestibility and amino acid content but, unfortunately, many are higher in salt and phosphorus than the older pet really needs.

Offer your dog a yummy Carrot Bone™ to help strengthen his teeth and gums. They are completely edible and irresistible to dogs.

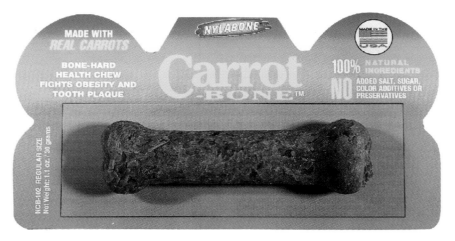

Older dogs are also more prone to developing arthritis and therefore it is important not to overfeed them since obesity puts added stress on the joints. For animals with joint pain, supplementing the diet with fatty acid combinations containing cis-linoleic acid, gamma-linolenic acid and eicosapentaenoic acid can be quite beneficial.

MEDICAL CONDITIONS AND DIET

Fat supplements are probably the most common supplements purchased from pet supply stores. They frequently promise to add luster, gloss, and sheen to the coat, and consequently make dogs look healthy. The only fatty acid that is essential for this purpose is cis-linoleic acid, which is found in flaxseed oil, sunflower seed oil, and safflower oil. Corn oil is a suitable but less effective alternative. Most of the other oils found in retail supplements are high in saturated and monounsaturated fats and are not beneficial for shiny fur or healthy skin. For dogs with allergies, arthritis, high blood pressure (hypertension), high cholesterol, and some heart ailments, other fatty acids may be prescribed by a veterinarian. The important ingredients in these

Although puppies need a diet of growth, the goal of an adult diet is one of maintenance.

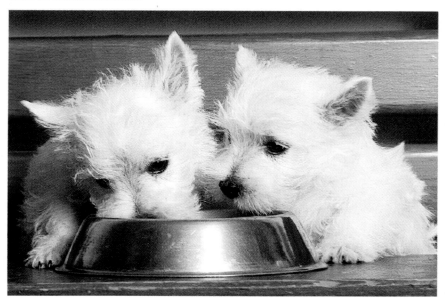

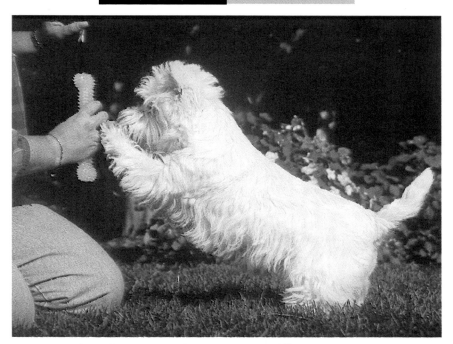

Let your dog chew on a Plaque Attacker™ Dental Bone, designed specifically to aid in the fight against periodontal disease.

products are gamma-linolenic acid (GLA), eicosapentaenoic acid (EPA), and docosahexaenoic acid (DHA). These products have gentle and natural anti-inflammatory properties. But don't be fooled by imitations. Most retail fatty acid supplements do not contain these functional forms of the essential fatty acids—look for gamma-linolenic acid, eicosapentaenoic acid, and docosahexaenoic acid on the label.

Zinc is an important mineral when it comes to immune function and wound healing but it has some other uses in the West Highland White Terrier. Zinc administration, particularly zinc acetate, can also promote copper excretion from the body. Usually this is not necessary or even desirable, but some West Highland White Terriers have an inherited disease that causes them to store copper in their liver; the result can be chronic hepatitis.

Although this copper-induced hepatitis cannot be cured, zinc supplementation can be used as a safe and effective form of therapy.

HEALTH

**PREVENTIVE MEDICINE AND HEALTH CARE
FOR YOUR WEST HIGHLAND WHITE TERRIER**

Keeping your West Highland White Terrier healthy requires preventive health care. This is not only the most effective but the least expensive way to battle illness. Good preventive care starts even before pup- 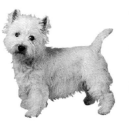 pies are born. The dam should be well cared for, vaccinated and free of infections and parasites.

Facing page: Regular visits to your veterinarian and good preventive health care will help your West Highland White Terrier live a long and happy life. Make sure your pet receives all the required vaccinations throughout his life.

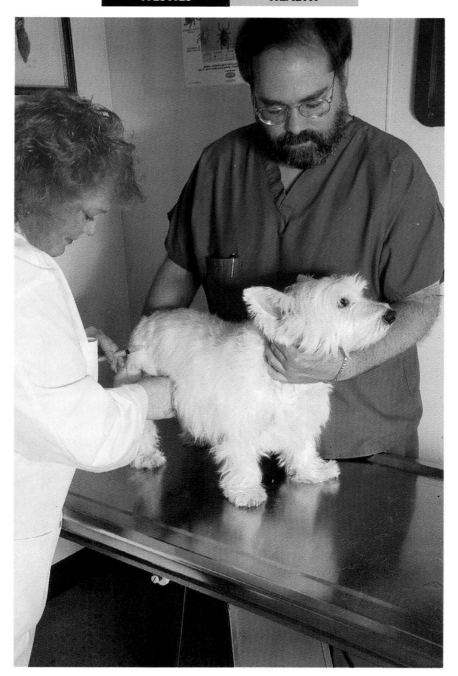

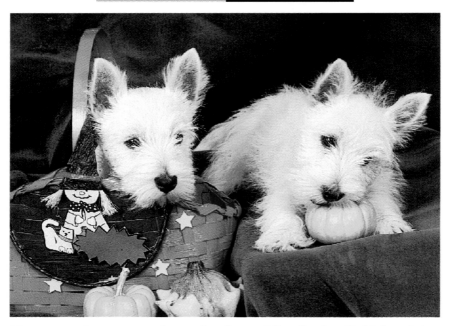

These puppies may not be such a "treat" for the family if they have worms. Assume that all puppies potentially have worms and institute worm control early.

Hopefully, both parents were screened for important genetic diseases (e.g. von Willebrands's disease), registered with the appropriate agencies (e.g., OFA, GDC, CERF), showed no evidence of medical or behavioral problems and were found to be good candidates for breeding. This gives the pup a good start in life. If all has been planned well, the dam will pass on resistance to disease to her pups that will last for the first few months of life. However, the dam can also pass on parasites, infections, genetic diseases and more.

TWO TO THREE WEEKS OF AGE

By two to three weeks of life, it is usually necessary to start pups on a regimen to control worms. Although dogs benefit from this parasite control, the primary reason for doing this is human health. After whelping, the dam often sheds large numbers of worms even if she tested negative previously. This is because many worms lay dormant in tissues and the stress of delivery causes parasite release and shedding into the environment. Assume that all puppies potentially have worms because studies have shown that 75% do. Thus, we institute worm control early to protect the people in the house from worms, more than the pups themselves. The deworming is repeated every two to three weeks until your veterinarian feels the condition is under control. Nursing bitches should be treated at the same time because they often shed worms during this time. Only use products recommended by your veterinarian. Over-the-counter parasiticides have been responsible for deaths in pups.

SIX TO TWENTY WEEKS OF AGE

Most puppies are weaned from their mother at six to eight weeks of age. Weaning shouldn't be done too early so that pups have the opportunity to socialize with their littermates and dam. This is important for them to be able to respond to other dogs later in life. There is no reason to rush the weaning process unless the dam can't produce enough milk to feed the pups.

Pups are usually first examined by their veterinarian at six

These happy, healthy puppies are nibbling on a Nylafloss™, which acts as dental floss for their teeth.

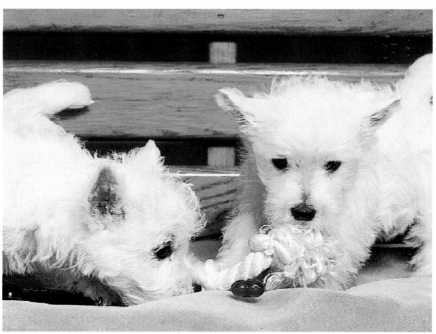

to eight weeks of age, which is when most vaccination schedules commence. If pups are exposed to many other dogs at this young age, veterinarians often opt for vaccinating with inactivated parvovirus at six weeks of age. When exposure isn't a factor, most veterinarians would rather wait to see the pup at eight weeks of age. At this point, they can also do a preliminary dental evaluation to see that all the puppy teeth are coming in correctly, check to see that the testicles are properly descending in males and that there are no health reasons to prohibit vaccination at this time. Heart murmurs, wandering knee-caps (luxating patellae), juvenile cataracts, persistent pupillary membranes (a congenital eye disease) and hernias are usually evident by this time.

Your veterinarian may also be able to perform temperament testing on the pup by eight weeks of age, or recommend someone to do it for you. Although temperament testing is not completely accurate, it can often predict which pups are most anxious and fearful. Some form of temperament evaluation is important because behavioral problems account for more animals being euthanized (killed) each year than all medical conditions combined.

Recently, some veterinary hospitals have been recommending neutering pups as early as six to eight weeks of age. A study done at the University of Florida College of Veterinary Medicine over a span of more than four years concluded there was no increase in complications when animals were neutered when less than six months of age. The evaluators also concluded that the surgery appeared to be less stressful when done in young pups.

Most vaccination schedules consist of injections being given at 6-8, 10-12 and 14-16 weeks of age. Ideally, vaccines should not be given closer than two weeks apart and three to four weeks seems to be optimal. Each vaccine usually consists of several different viruses (e.g., parvovirus, distemper, parainfluenza, hepatitis) combined into one injection. Coronavirus can be given as a separate vaccination according to this same schedule if pups are at risk. Some veterinarians and breeders advise another parvovirus booster at 18-20 weeks of age. A booster is given for all vaccines at one year of age and annually thereafter. For animals at increased risk of exposure, parvovirus vaccination may be given as often as four times a year. A new vaccine for canine cough (tracheobronchitis) is squirted into the nostrils. It can be given as early as six weeks of age if pups are at risk. Leptospirosis vaccination is given in some geographic areas and likely offers protection for 6-8 months. The initial series consists of three to four injections spaced two to three weeks apart, starting as early as 10 weeks of age. Rabies vaccine is given as a separate injection at three months of age, then repeated when the pup is one year old, then every one to three years depending up local risk and government regulation.

Between 8 and 14 weeks of age, use every opportunity to expose the pup to as many people and situations as possible. This is part of the critical socialization period that will determine how good a pet your dog will become. This is not the time to abandon a puppy for eight hours while you go to work. This is also not the time to punish your dog in any way, shape or form.

This is the time to introduce your dog to neighborhood cats, birds and other creatures. Hold off on exposure to other dogs until after the second vaccination in the series. You don't want your new friend to pick up con-

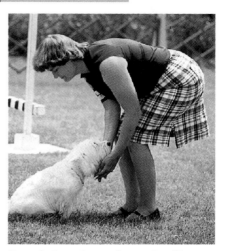

Participating in obedience classes—and going on to compete—helps to properly socialize your Westie because it introduces the dog to many different people and situations. The more varied the exposure, the better the socialization.

tagious diseases from dogs it meets in its travels before it has adequate protection. By 12 weeks of age, your pup should be ready for social outings with other dogs. Do them—they're a great way for your dog to feel comfortable around members of its own species. Walk the streets and introduce your pup to everybody you meet. Your goal should be to introduce your dog to every type of person or situation it is likely to encounter in its life. Take it in cars, elevators, buses, travel crates, subways, parade grounds, beaches; you want it to habituate to all environments. Expose your pup to kids, teenagers, old people, people in wheelchairs, people on bicycles, people in uniforms. The more varied the exposure, the better the socialization.

Proper identification of your pet is also important since this minimizes the risk of theft and increases the chances that your pet will be returned to you if it is lost. There are several different options. Microchip implantation is a relatively painless procedure involving the subcutaneous injection of an implant the

A thorough examination by your veterinarian is necessary to ensure your pet is in tip-top condition.

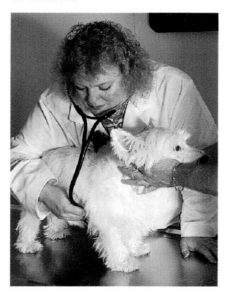

size of a grain of rice. This implant does not act as a beacon if your pet goes missing. However, if your pet turns up at a veterinary clinic or shelter and is checked with a scanner, the chip provides information about the owner that can be used to quickly reunite you with your pet. This method of identification is reasonably priced, permanent in nature, and performed at most veterinary clinics. Another option is tattooing which can be done on the inner ear or on the skin of the abdomen. Most purebreds are given a number by the associated registry (e.g., American Kennel Club, United Kennel Club, Canadian Kennel Club, etc.) and this is used for identification. Alternatively, permanent numbers such as social security numbers (telephone numbers and addresses may change during the life of your pet) can be used in the tattooing process. There are several different tattoo registries maintaining lists of dogs, their tattoo codes and their owners. Finally, identifying collars and tags provide quick information but can be separated from your pet if it is lost of stolen. They work best when combined with a permanent identification system such as microchip implantation or tattoo.

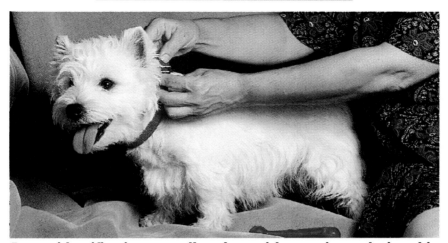

Proper identification on a collar, along with tattooing and microchip implanting, will increase the chances of being reunited with your Westie should you become separated.

FOUR TO TWELVE MONTHS OF AGE

At 16 weeks of age, when your pup gets the last in its series of regular induction vaccinations, ask your veterinarian about evaluating the pup for hip dysplasia with the PennHip™ technique. Since anesthesia is typically required for the procedure, many veterinarians like to do the evaluation at the same time as neutering.

At this same time, it is very worthwhile to perform a diagnostic test for von Willebrand's disease, an inherited disorder that causes uncontrolled bleeding. A simple blood test is all that is required, but it may need to be sent to a special laboratory to have the test performed.

As a general rule, neuter your animal at about six months of age unless you fully intend to breed it. As mentioned earlier, neutering can be safely done at eight weeks of age but this is still not a common practice. Neutering not only stops the possibility of pregnancy and undesirable behaviors, but can prevent several health problems as well. It is a well established fact that pups spayed before their first heat have a dramatically reduced incidence of mammary (breast) cancer. Neutered males significantly decrease their incidence of prostate disorders.

Also when your pet is six months of age, your veterinarian will want to take a blood sample to perform a heartworm

43

test. If the test is negative and shows no evidence of heartworm infection, the pup will go on heartworm prevention therapy. Some veterinarians are even recommending preventive therapy in younger pups. This might be a one-a-day regimen, but newer therapies can be given on a once-a-month basis. As a bonus, most of these heartworm preventatives also help prevent internal parasites (worms, as mentioned above).

Another part of the six month visit should be a thorough dental evaluation to make sure all the permanent teeth have correctly erupted. If they haven't, this will be the time to correct the problem. Correction should only be performed to make the animal more comfortable and promote more normal chewing. The procedures should never be used to cosmetically improve the appearance of a dog used for show purposes or breeding.

After the dental evaluation, you should start implementing home dental care. In most cases, this will consist of brushing the teeth one or more times each week and perhaps using dental rinses. It is a sad fact that 85% of dogs over four years of age have periodontal disease and doggy breath. In fact it is so common that most people think it is "nor-

mal." Well, it is normal—as normal as bad breath would be in people if they never brushed their teeth. Brush your dog's teeth regularly with a special tooth brush and toothpaste and you can greatly reduce the incidence of tartar buildup, bad breath and gum disease. Better preventive care means that dogs live a long time. They'll enjoy their sunset years more if they still have their teeth. Ask your veterinarian for details on home dental care.

ONE TO SEVEN YEARS OF AGE

At one year of age, your dog should be re-examined again and have boosters for all vaccines. Your veterinarian will also want to do a very thorough physical examination to look for early evidence of problems. This might include taking radiographs (x-rays) of the hips and elbows to look for evidence of dysplastic changes. Genetic Disease Control (GDC) will certify hips and elbows at 12 months of age; Orthopedic Foundation for Animals won't issue certification until 24 months of age. The West Highland White Terrier now has a relatively low incidence of both hip and elbow dysplasia.

At 12 months of age, it's also a great time to have some blood samples analyzed to provide background information. It is a good idea to have baseline levels of thyroid hormones (free and total), blood cell counts, it's time for another veterinary visit. This visit is a wonderful opportunity for a thorough clinical examination rather than just "shots". Since 85% of dogs have

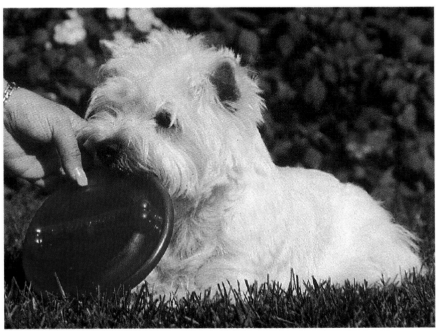

Implement home dental care by giving your Westie a Gumabone® Frisbee™ to gnaw on. It will provide hours of fun as well as keep your pet's teeth strong and healthy. The trademark Frisbee is used under license from Mattel, Inc., California, USA.

organ chemistries, and cholesterol levels. This can serve as a valuable comparison to samples collected in the future. It may also help identify those Westies that develop liver disease (hepatitis) due to copper accumulation.

Each year, preferably around the time of your pet's birthday, periodontal disease by four years of age, veterinary intervention does not seem to be as widespread as it should be. The examination should include visually inspecting the ears, eyes (a great time to start scrutinizing for progressive retinal atrophy, cataracts, etc.), mouth (don't wait for gum disease), and groin,

45

listening (auscultation) to the lungs and heart, feeling (palpating) the lymph nodes and abdomen and answering all of your questions about optimal health care. In addition, booster vaccinations are given during these times, feces are checked for parasites, urine is analyzed and blood samples may be collected for analysis. One of the tests run on the blood sample is for heartworm antigen. In areas of the country where heartworm is only present in the spring, summer and fall (it's spread by mosquitoes), blood samples are collected and evaluated about a month prior to the mosquito season. Other routine blood tests are for blood cells (hematology), organ chemistries, thyroid levels and electrolytes.

By two years of age, most veterinarians prefer to begin preventive dental cleanings, often referred to as "prophies." Anesthesia is required and the veterinarian or veterinary dentist will use an ultrasonic scaler to remove plaque and tartar from above and below the gum line and polish the teeth so that plaque has a harder time sticking to the teeth. Radiographs (x-rays) and fluoride treatments are other options. It is now known that it is plaque, not tartar, that initiates inflammation in the gums. Since scaling and root planing remove more tartar than plaque, veterinary dentists have begun using a new technique called PerioBUD (Periodontal Bactericidal Ultrasonic Debridement). The ultrasonic treatment is quicker, disrupts more bacteria and is less irritating to the gums. With tooth polishing to finish up the procedure, gum healing is better and owners can start home care sooner. Each dog has its own dental needs that must be addressed, but most veterinary dentists recommend prophies annually.

SENIOR WEST HIGHLAND WHITE TERRIERS

West Highland White Terriers are considered seniors when they reach about seven to nine years of age. Veterinarians still usually only need to examine them once a year, but it is now important to start screening for geriatric problems. Accordingly blood profiles, urinalysis, chest radiographs (x-rays) and electrocardiograms (EKG) are recommended on an annual basis. When problems are caught early, they are much more likely to be successfully managed. This is as true in canine medicine as it is in human medicine.

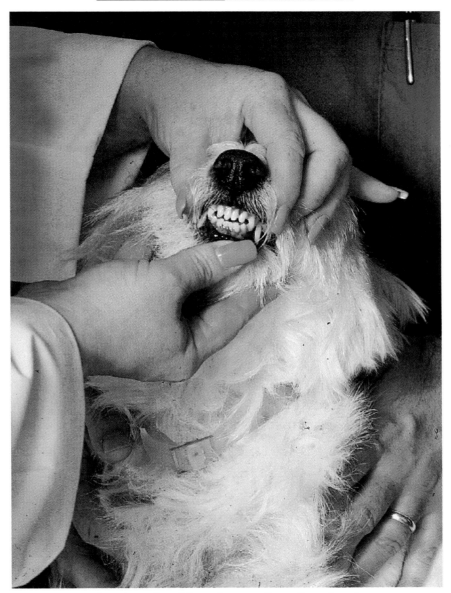

Your veterinarian should perform a dental evaluation on your dog at six months of age to make sure all the permanent teeth have come in correctly. By two years of age, most vets like to begin preventive dental cleanings called "prophies."

MEDICAL PROBLEMS

RECOGNIZED GENETIC CONDITIONS SPECIFICALLY RELATED TO THE WEST HIGHLAND WHITE TERRIER

Many conditions appear to be especially prominent in West Highland White Terriers. Sometimes it is possible to identify the genetic basis of a problem, but in many cases, we must be satisfied with merely identifying the breeds that are at risk and how the conditions can be identified,

Facing page: As a responsible West Highland White Terrier owner, you should have a basic understanding of the medical problems that affect the breed. This is Judy Arenz's Ch. Lor-E-L's Snickers Bar-None.

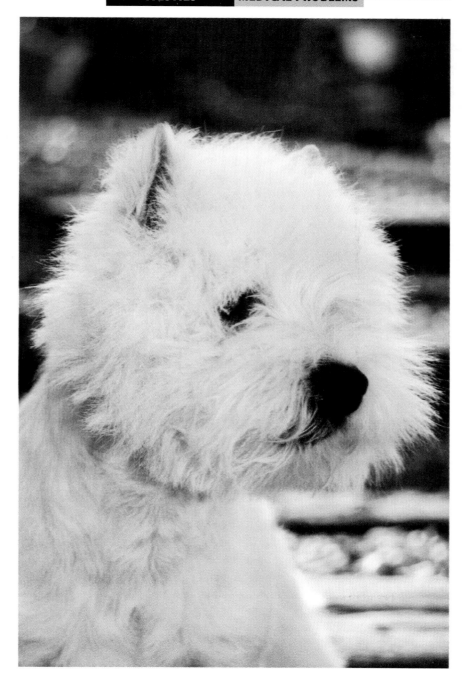

treated and prevented. Following are some conditions that have been recognized as being common in the West Highland White Terrier but this listing is certainly not complete. Also, many genetic conditions may be common in certain breed lines, not in the breed in general.

CATARACTS

Cataracts refer to an opacity or cloudiness on the lens and ophthalmologists are careful to categorize them on the basis of stage, age of onset, and location. In Westies, cataracts can be inherited as an autosomal recessive trait (with variable expressivity) meaning that both parents need carry the trait for pups to be affected. The cataracts are usually evident quite early, often in young pups but almost always before one year of age. These congenital cataracts are nuclear and cortical, progressive in nature and may be associated with microphthalmia (smaller than normal eyes). Westies are also prone to juvenile cataracts located at the posteriorY suture which are nonprogressive in nature. Many dogs adapt well to cataracts, but cataract removal surgery is available and quite successful if needed. The condition may be associated with persistent hyperplastic primary vitreous as discussed below. Affected animals and their siblings should obviously not be used for breeding and careful ophthalmologic evaluation of both parents is warranted.

CRANIOMANDIBULAR OSTEOPATHY

Craniomandibular osteopathy is a bizarre proliferative bone disease that typically affects the lower jawbone (mandible), the tympanic bullae of the inner ear, and, occasionally, other bones of the head. The cause is unknown but clearly the condition is not cancerous or inflammatory, although it certainly appears that way. Affected animals are typically less than one year of age.

The condition does not cause clinical problems in all cases. However, affected animals often have difficulty chewing and swallowing and may experience some pain when opening their mouths. The diagnosis is usually suspected when a young dog of a breed at risk, such as a West Highland White Terrier, experiences the clinical signs listed above. The diagnosis is confirmed by radiography (x-rays) in which selected bones of the head show thickening associated with proliferation of bone. Ra-

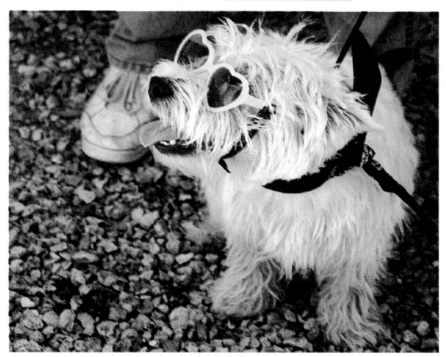

Behind his "cool" shades, this Westie's eyes are clear and dark. Any redness or cloudiness could indicate a problem and should be examined immediately by your veterinarian. Owners, Lelia Livengood and Daphne Gentry.

diographs should be repeated every three months to monitor progression or regression of the condition. Blood profiles of affected dogs may demonstrate increased serum calcium levels and some enzymes such as serum alkaline phosphatase.

There are no effective therapies available, but luckily the condition is often self-limiting. The abnormal bone growth slows, often stops, and may even recede by about a year of age. In the interim, symptomatic therapy consists of anti-inflammatory therapy (e.g., aspirin), feeding soft foods, and perhaps tube feeding if opening the mouth is painful. Sometimes euthanasia is necessary if animals can't eat and are in much pain. Affected animals should not be used for breeding, even if they recover completely.

ELBOW DYSPLASIA
Elbow dysplasia and osteoch-

ondrosis are disorders of young dogs, with problems usually starting between four and seven months of age. The usual manifestation is a sudden onset of lameness. In time, the continued inflammation results in arthritis in those affected joints.

West Highland White Terriers are not particularly prone to elbow dysplasia and, since the incidence is so low, continued registration is recommended because it should be possible to completely eliminate the condition in Westies by conscientious breeding. Radiographs (x-rays) are taken of the elbow joints and submitted to a registry for evaluation. The Orthopedic Foundation for Animals (OFA) will assign a breed registry number to those animals with normal elbows that are over 24 months of age. Genetic Disease Control for Animals (GDC) maintains an open registry for elbow dysplasia and assigns a registry number to those individuals with normal elbows at 12 months of age or older. Only animals with "normal" elbows should be used for breeding.

EPIDERMAL DYSPLASIA

Epidermal dysplasia is a developmental skin problem seen most commonly in the West Highland White Terrier. Affected pups are often itchy, their skin becomes dark and thickened, and in many ways they look like severely allergic pups, only younger than usual. Likely because of the accumulation of surface scale, there is commonly an associated yeast infection with the organism *Malassezia pachydermatis*. The condition can get bad enough that some breeders have referred to affected individuals as "armadillo Westies".

The diagnosis is made on the basis of skin biopsies and it is important that the pathology samples be interpreted by someone with expertise in skin problems since the characteristic changes can be subtle. Yeast organisms might also be seen on these samples as surface parasites. Treatment must be very intensive using topical preparations and strong oral medications. Selenium disulfide or chlorhexidine shampoos are used to help control yeast and rehydrate the skin, which tends to be dry but greasy. In most instances, vitamin A-derived medications such as etretinate are prescribed to attempt to control the excessive scale formation. The goal is to control the situation; no cures are known. Affected animals and their immediate relatives should not be used for breeding.

GLAUCOMA

Glaucoma is one of the leading causes of blindness in animals and is caused by an increase in fluid pressure within the eye. Anything that interferes with the drainage of fluid inside the eye can result in glaucoma and not all have a genetic basis. However, primary glaucoma does occur in several breeds, including the Westie. There are three distinct types of inherited glaucoma: open-angle (as seen in West Highland White Terriers); narrow-angle (as seen in Cocker Spaniels and Miniature Poodles), and; goniodysgenesis as seen in American Cocker Spaniels and Chow Chows.

With glaucoma, the eyes are often red and painful. Most Westies are over five years of age when first affected and the problem is often associated with the infiltration of pigment cells (melanocytosis). The diagnosis is confirmed with a tonometer that measures the pressure within the eye. Gonioscopy is a technique used to visually inspect the drainage angle within the eye and determine the exact cause of the problem. Treatment can involve medical or surgical options depending on the severity of the disorder. Hereditary glaucoma can be prevented by screening all animals

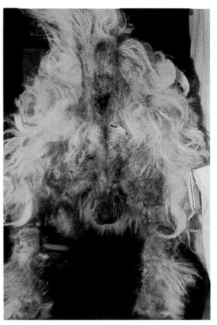

Westies are prone to developmental skin problems such as epidermal dysplasia that can cause their skin to look dark and scaly and become extremely itchy.

used in breeding programs.

GLOBOID CELL LEUKODYSTROPHY (GCL)

Globoid Cell Leukodystrophy is a lysosomal storage disease most commonly reported in the West Highland White Terrier and the Cairn Terrier. It is a neurological disease associated with an inherited (autosomal recessive) lack of the critical enzyme galactocerebromide-b-galactosidase. Researchers at the Jefferson

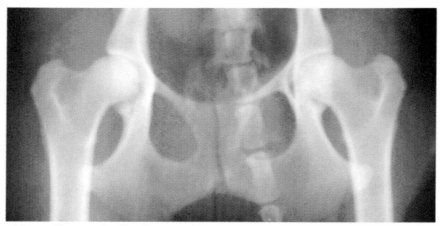

This radiograph displays a dog that recieved an OFA "excellent" when x-rayed for hip dysplasia. Both of the hip joints are clear of dysplasia.

Medical College's Division of Medical Genetics, as part of their research on the human condition, have determined the gene mutation responsible. Affected animals appear normal at birth but fail to develop normally with their littermates. The enzyme defect results in alterations in the cerebrum and cerebellum and problems are usually evident by 11-30 weeks of age. Animals tend to develop tremors, stilted gait, muscle weakness and even behavioral changes. The course is progressive and invariably fatal. Both parents should be presumed to be carriers and not used in further breedings. The carrier state can be detected by submitting a blood sample in a heparinized tube to the GLC researchers at the Jefferson Medical College, 1100 Walnut Street, Room 410, Philadelphia, P.A. 19107. A commercial test available from veterinary laboratories is not yet available.

HIP DYSPLASIA

Hip dysplasia is a genetically transmitted developmental problem of the hip joint that is common in many breeds. Happily, it is relatively rare in the West Highland White Terrier. Dogs may be born with a "susceptibility" or "tendency" to develop hip dysplasia but it is not a foregone conclusion that all susceptible dogs will eventually develop hip dysplasia. All dysplastic dogs are born with normal hips and the dysplastic

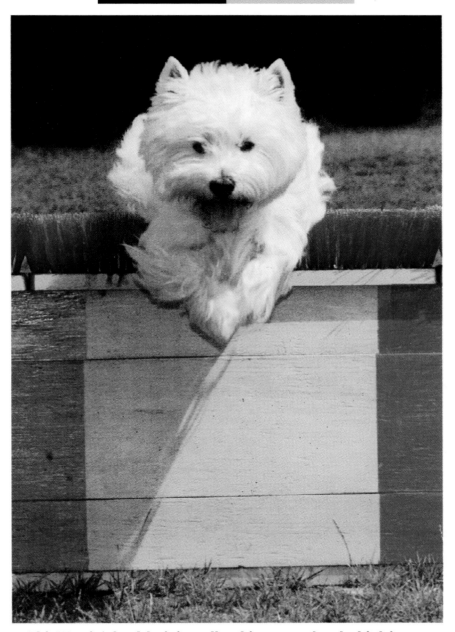

This Westie's healthy joints allow him to excel at the high jump.
This flier is Lucky Lord Floyd owned by H. Valentijn.

changes begin within the first 24 months of life although they are usually evident long before then.

When purchasing a West Highland White Terrier pup, it is best to ensure that the parents were both registered with normal hips through one of the international registries such as the Orthopedic Foundation for Animals or Genetic Disease Control. Pups over 16 weeks of age can be tested by veterinarians trained in the PennHip™ procedure, which is a way of predicting risk of developing hip dysplasia and arthritis. In time it should be possible to completely eradicate hip dysplasia from the breed.

Hair loss is a symptom of many different conditions, including hypothyroidism, epidermal dysplasia and allergies.

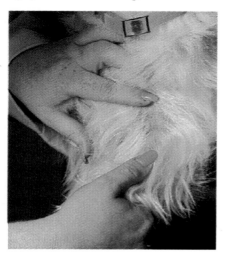

HYPOTHYROIDISM

Hypothyroidism is the most commonly diagnosed endocrine (hormonal) problem in the West Highland White Terrier. The disease itself refers to an insufficient amount of thyroid hormones being produced. In most cases, affected animals appear fine until they use up most of their remaining thyroid hormone reserves. The most common manifestations then are lack of energy and recurrent infections. Hair loss is seen in about one-third of cases.

You might suspect that hypothyroidism would be easy to diagnose but it is trickier than you think. Since there is a large reserve of thyroid hormones in the body, a test measuring only total blood levels of the hormones (T-4 and T-3) is not a very sensitive indicator of the condition. Thyroid stimulation tests are the best way to measure the functional reserve. Measuring "free" and "total" levels of the hormones or endogenous TSH (thyroid stimulating hormone) are other approaches. Fortunately, although there may be some problems in diagnosing hypothyroidism, treatment is straightforward and relatively inexpensive. Supplementing the affected animal twice daily with thyroid hormone effectively

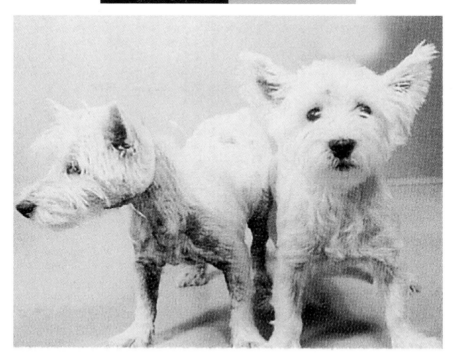

Inhalant allergies are very common in the West Highland White Terrier. These two pups are suffering from skin rashes and infections.

treats the condition. Animals with hypothyroidism should not be used in a breeding program and those with circulating autoantibodies but no actual hypothyroid disease should also not be used for breeding.

INHALANT ALLERGIES

Inhalant allergy is the canine version of hay fever and is extremely common, especially in the West Highland White Terrier. Whereas people with allergies often sneeze, dogs with allergies scratch–they're itchy. The most common manifestations include licking and chewing at the front feet. There may also be face rubbing, a rash on the belly or in the armpits and subsequent bacterial infections on the skin surface. Allergic Westies also seem to quickly develop skin thickness and the skin color changes quickly from red to black with the ensuing inflammation.

The offenders are molds, pollens and house dust that are present in the air. Most pollen allergies are seasonal but house dust and mold allergies are usually present throughout the year. Most dogs start to have problems some time after six months of age. This is an important distinction because epidermal dysplasia looks quite similar but typically starts prior to six months of age.

Allergies are diagnosed in dogs similar to the way they are diagnosed in people. Intradermal (skin) testing is the most specific test and is usually done by veterinary dermatologists or others in referral settings. To perform the test, we shave a rectangular area on their side for the test site and the potentially allergy-causing substances (allergens) are injected individu-

ally. It is not unusual to test for 40 or more allergens during an allergy test and the site has to be large enough to accommodate one injection for each allergen. In the Westie, this usually amounts to the entire side of the chest. The procedure is relatively painless since only a very tiny amount is actually injected, and with a very small needle, and only into the very uppermost layers of the skin. It is best to test Westies early, before their skin gets too thickened and dark. This greatly complicates the interpretation of the skin tests. Blood tests are also available for allergy testing but are, at present, less reliable. However, they are

Certain molds and pollens found outside can cause an allergic reaction in your dog. Watch your Westie carefully for any signs of irritation or scratching when playing outdoors.

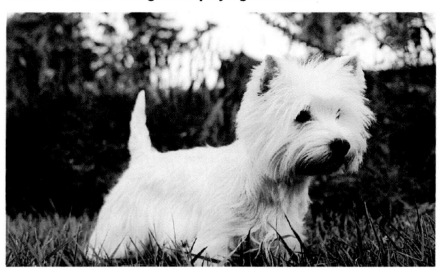

the most suitable when allergies have been going on for a while and the skin is too thickened or inflamed for reliable skin testing.

Mild cases of allergy can be treated with antihistamines, fatty acid supplements (combinations of eicosapentaenoic acid and gamma-linolenic acid) and frequent soothing baths. Allergies that last for more than three or four months each year or are severe are best treated with immunotherapy (allergy shots). In fact, in the West Highland White Terrier, it is advisable to skin test early and start animals on immunotherapy without delay. Corticosteroids effectively reduce the itch of allergy but can cause other medical problems with long-term use.

One of the quickest ways to comfort an allergic pet is with a relaxing bath. The effect doesn't last long but it does help to relieve itchiness. The bath water should be cool rather than hot since hot water can actually make the itchiness worse. Adding colloidal oatmeal powder or Epsom salts to the bath water makes it even more soothing and a variety of medicated shampoos available from veterinarians will also improve the situation. It is unlikely that a medicated bath will reduce itchi-

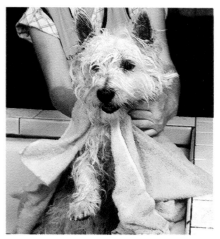

One of the best ways to soothe an allergic Westie is to give him a cool bath with Epsom salts or oatmeal powder. This dog certainly looks refreshed and relaxed!

ness for more than a couple of days but it is a safe way to give your allergic pet some relief and it can be repeated frequently. There are many safe sprays available from your veterinarian that can also give some temporary relief. If the allergies are complicated by infection, the infection may also be itchy; antibiotics are sometimes required.

The only effective way of preventing inhalant allergies is to select pups from parents that aren't allergic themselves. This is a complicated process since animals may be bred before they are old enough to show evidence of allergies.

LEGG-CALVE-PERTHES DISEASE

Legg-Calve-Perthes Disease is a disorder of the hip joint seen in young, small-breed dogs. It is also known as aseptic necrosis of the femoral head. Typically it is seen in dogs between four and twelve months of age and only one leg is affected in the majority (85%) of cases. A genetic trend has been suggested, involving an autosomal recessive trait with incomplete penetrance.

Affected dogs are typically lame on one leg and in great pain. There may be substantial atrophy of muscle in the affected area. The diagnosis can be suspected on the basis of radiographs (x-rays) but surgical biopsies are needed for confirmation. Treatment involves surgically removing the damaged femoral head. Since most cases occur in small dogs that aren't bearing a lot of weight on the hip joint, further reconstructive surgery is not usually necessary. The Institute for Genetic Disease Control in Animals (GDC) has plans for provide an open registry for this condition. It should thus be possible to select animals with no family history of Legg-Calve-Perthes Disease and hopefully eliminate the trait from the gene pool.

LIVER DISEASE DUE TO COPPER ACCUMULATION

Some dogs are prone to developing liver disease in association with an inherited metabolic defect which causes copper to accumulate in the liver and lead to toxicity. This is similar to Wilson's Disease in people. The West Highland White Terrier is not the breed affected most often (that would be the Bedlington Terrier), but the incidence is high enough to warrant mention here. The condition is spread as a recessive trait so both parents must be carriers if a dog is found to be affected.

Affected dogs develop a slowly-progressive form of liver disease. They are usually in young adulthood when the condition is first recognized. Jaundice only develops late in the course of the disease when liver function is severely compromised.

Very recently, researchers have discovered a genetic marker for copper toxicosis that can be detected by a blood test. Although not yet widely available as a commercial test, this laboratory evaluation is an exceptionally important method for detecting carriers of the disease. Those carriers should be removed from all breeding possibilities and then it should be

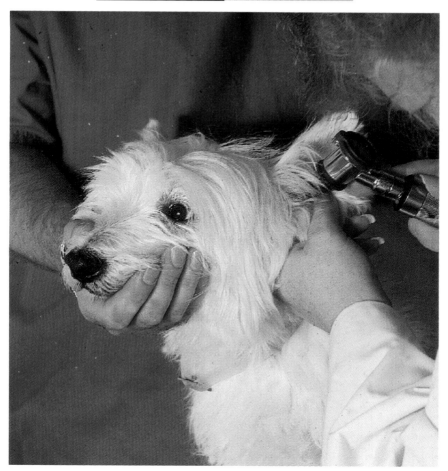

Your veterinarian will check your Westie's ears for any signs of infection or waxy build-up.

possible to completely eliminate the trait in West Highland White Terriers.

MEDIAL PATELLAR LUXATION

The patella is the kneecap and patellar luxation refers to the condition when the knee-cap slips out of its usual resting place and lodges on the inside (medial aspect) of the knee. It is a congenital problem of dogs but the degree of patellar displacement may increase with time as the tissues stretch and the bones continue to deform. The condition is seen primarily in small and toy breeds of dogs.

Medial patellar luxation may be graded by veterinarians as to how much laxity there is in the patella. No laxity is preferred and affected individuals may have Grade I (mild) through Grade IV (severe). The diagnosis can be made by manipulating the knee joint to see if the kneecap luxates towards the inner (medial) aspect of the leg. There is usually little or no pain associated with this process. Radiograph's (x-rays) can be used to document persistent luxation and to evaluate for other abnormalities such as arthritic changes.

Older dogs and those mildly affected may respond to conservative therapy, but surgery is often recommended for young dogs before arthritic changes become evident. There are several successful surgical techniques for this condition. After surgery, dogs should have enforced rest for six weeks while healing, and leash activity only. The results are excellent in most cases.

The best form of prevention is to only purchase animals that have no family history of medial patellar luxation. Registries are maintained by the Orthopedic Foundation for Animals (OFA) and the Institute for Genetic Disease Control in Animals (GDC).

PULMONIC STENOSIS

Pulmonic stenosis refers to a stricture or incomplete opening through the pulmonic valve within the heart. The valve is located between the right ventricle and the pulmonary artery, which delivers the blood from the heart to the lungs. Many dogs with pulmonic stenosis are asymptomatic but do have a hear murmur. As they get older or if the condition is severe, there may be evidence of exercise intolerance, fainting (syncope), coughing, or fluid accumulation within the body.

An accurate diagnosis of pulmonic stenosis is made by the use of physical examination, radiographs (x-rays), electrocardiogram, (EKG) and either echocardiogram (ultrasound examination of the heart) or cardiac catheterization. Quite often it is necessary to inject a medical dye solution during a catheterization of the heart to visualize the defect on a series of radiographs. This is known as an angiogram.

Many cases of pulmonic stenosis are mild and don't require therapy. More severe blockages will result in heart failure and therefore require corrective surgery. Affected animals should not be used in breeding programs.

VON WILLEBRAND'S DISEASE

Von Willebrand's disease (vWD) is the most common inherited bleeding disorder of dogs. The abnormal gene can be inherited from one or both parents. If both parents pass on the gene, most of the resultant pups fail to thrive and most will die. In most cases, though, the pup inherits a relative lack of clotting ability which is quite variable. For instance, one dog may have 15% of the clotting factor, while another might have 60%. The higher the amount, the less likely it will be that the bleeding will be readily evident since spontaneous bleeding is usually only seen when dogs have less than

Genetic diseases can be passed to Westie puppies from their parents. It is important to identify these problems before breeding in order to ensure healthy animals.

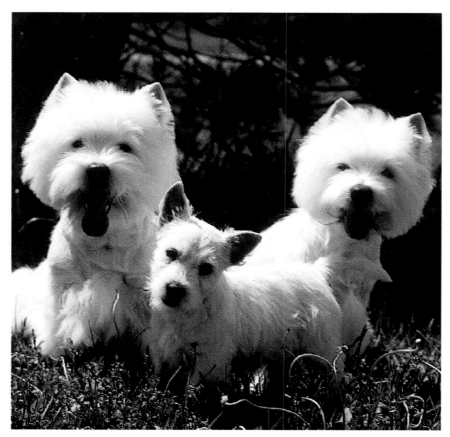

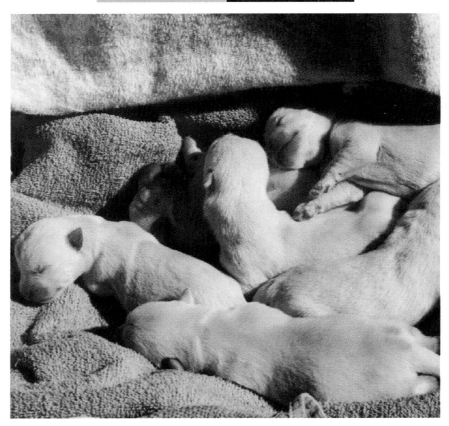

Von Willebrand's disease is just one of the many conditions that can be passed genetically from parents to puppies. Your puppy's veterinarian can check his blood to test for sufficient von Willebrand factor.

30% of the normal level of von Willebrand clotting factor. Thus, some dogs don't get diagnosed until they are neutered or spayed and they end up bleeding uncontrollably or they develop pockets of blood (hematomas) at the surgical site.

There are tests available to determine the amount of von Willebrand factor in the blood and they are accurate and reasonably priced. Westies used for breeding should have normal amounts of von Willebrand factor in their blood and so should all pups that are adopted as household pets. Carriers should not be used for breeding, even if they appear clinically normal.

OTHER CONDITIONS COMMONLY SEEN IN THE WEST HIGHLAND WHITE TERRIER

- Atrioventricular Block
- Cleft Palate
- Deafness
- Ichthyosis
- Inguinal Hernia
- Keratoconjunctivitis Sicca
- Lens Luxation
- Malassezia Dermatitis
- Mandibular Mesioclusion

- (underbite)
- Microphthalmia
- Myotonia (Congenital)
- Persistent Pupillary Membranes
- Pyruvate Kinase Deficiency
- Retained Primary Teeth
- Retinal Dysplasia (Retinal Folds)
- Seborrhea

Although your Westie may look the picture of health, there are many conditions that are not obvious to the eye. That is why regular veterinary check-ups are so important for good preventive care.

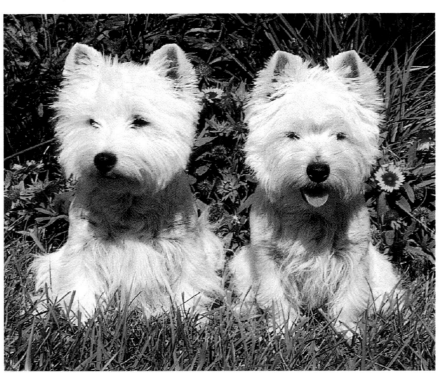

INFECTIONS &
INFESTATIONS

**HOW TO PROTECT YOUR WEST HIGHLAND WHITE
TERRIER FROM PARASITES AND MICROBES**

An important part of keeping your West Highland White Terrier healthy is to prevent problems caused by parasites and microbes. Although there are a variety of drugs available that can help limit problems, prevention is always the desired option. Taking the proper precautions leads to less itching and less expense.

Facing page: Understanding how to protect your West Highland White Terrier from infections and infestations is the best way to avoid any problems. Daphne Gentry and Betty Williams' Ch. Killundine Made In A Dandy Way looks flea-free!

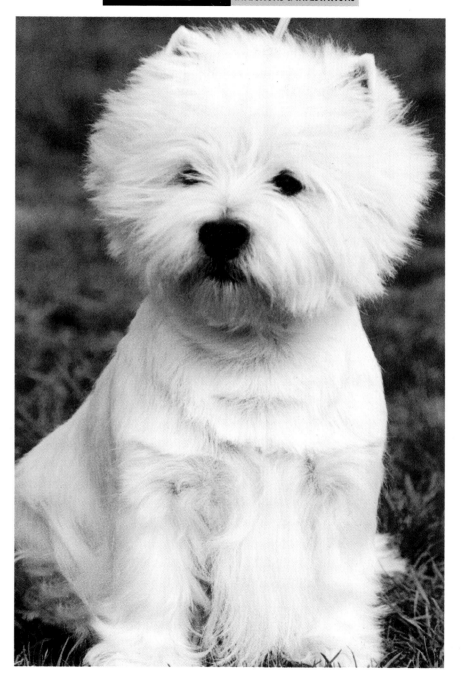

FLEAS

Fleas are important and common parasites but not an inevitable part of every pet owner's reality. If you take the time to understand some of the basics of flea population dynamics, control is both conceivable and practical.

Fleas have four life stages (egg, larva, pupa, adult) and each stage responds to some therapies while being resistant to others. Failing to understand this is the major reason why some people have so much trouble getting the upper hand in the battle to control fleas.

Fleas spend all their time on dogs and only leave if physically removed by brushing, bathing or scratching. However, the eggs that are laid on the animal are not sticky and fall to the ground to contaminate the environment. Our goal must be to remove fleas from the animals in the house, from the house itself and from the immediate outdoor environment. Part of our plan must also involve using different medications to get rid of

Dogs love to romp in the grass, but it is also one of the most common places to pick up parasites. Make sure you check your dog carefully for fleas and ticks after playing outdoors.

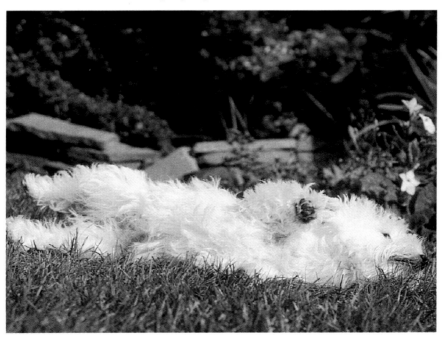

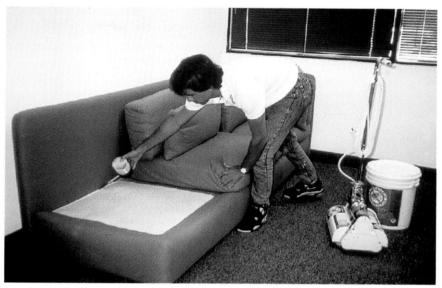

The best approach to prevent and eliminate flea infestation in the house is to use a safe insecticide to kill adult fleas in the house and then an insect growth regulator to stop the eggs and larvae in the environment.

the different life stages as well as minimizing the use of potentially harmful insecticides that could be poisonous for pets and family members.

A flea comb is a very handy device for recovering fleas from pets. The best places to comb are the tailhead, groin area, armpits, back and neck region. Fleas collected should be dropped into a container of alcohol which quickly kills them before they can escape. In addition, all pets should be bathed with a cleansing shampoo (or flea shampoo) to remove fleas and eggs. This has no residual effect, however,

and fleas can jump back on immediately after the bath if nothing else is done. Rather than using potent insecticidal dips and sprays, consider products containing the safe pyrethrins imidacloprid or fipronil, and the insect growth regulators (such as methoprene and pyripoxyfen or insect development inhibitors (IDIs) such as lufenuron. These products are not only extremely safe, but the combination is effective against eggs, larvae and adults. This only leaves the pupal stage to cause continued problems. Insect growth regulators can also be safely given as once-a-month oral preparations. Flea collars are rarely useful, and electronic flea collars are not to be recommended for any dogs.

To clean up the household, vacuuming is a good first step because it picks up about 50% of the flea eggs and it also stimulates flea pupae to emerge as adults, a stage when they are easier to kill with insecticides. The vacuum bag should then be removed and discarded with each treatment. Household treatment can then be initiated with pyrethrins and a combination of either insect growth regulars or sodium polyborate (a borax derivative). The pyre-thrins need to be reapplied every two to three weeks but the insect growth regulators last about two to three months and many companies guarantee sodium polyborate for a full year. Stronger insecticides such as carbamates and organophosphates can be used and will last three to four weeks in the household, but they are potentially toxic and offer no real advantages other than their persistence in the home environment. This is also one of their major disadvantages.

When an insecticide is combined with an insect growth regulator, flea control is most likely

The most effective way to prevent ticks is to remove underbrush and leaf litter. This eliminates the cover and food source for small mammals that serve as hosts.

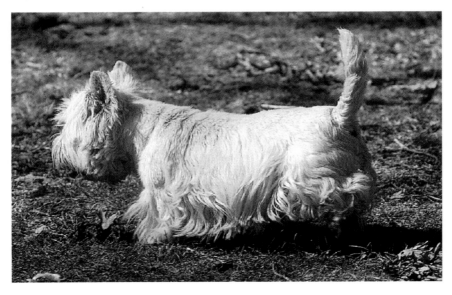

to be successful. The insecticide kills the adult fleas and the insect growth regulator affects the eggs and larvae. However, insecticides kill less that 20% of flea cocoons (pupae). Because of this, new fleas may hatch in two to three weeks despite appropriate application of products. This is known as the "pupal window" and is one of the most common causes for ineffective flea control. This is why a safe insecticide should be applied to the home environment two to three weeks after the initial treatment. This catches the newly hatched pupae before they have a chance to lay eggs and continue the flea problem.

If treatment of the outdoor environment is needed, there are several options. Pyripoxyfen, an insect growth regulator, is stable in sunlight and can be used outdoors. Sodium polyborate can be used as well, but it is important that it not be inadvertently eaten by pets. Organophosphates and carbamates are sometimes recommended for outdoor use and it is not necessary to treat the entire property. Flea control should be directed predominantly at garden margins, porches, dog houses, garages, and in other pet lounging areas. Fleas don't do well with direct exposure to sunlight so

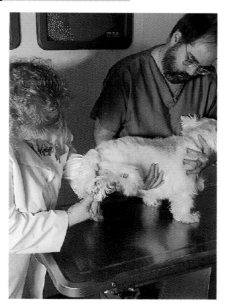

Ticks can climb up your dog from his feet, so check your Westie's paws after walking outside.

generalized lawn treatment is not needed. Finally, microscopic worms (nematodes) are available that can be sprayed onto the lawn with a garden sprayer. The nematodes eat immature flea forms and then biodegrade without harming anything else.

TICKS

Ticks are found world wide and can cause a variety of problems including blood loss, tick paralysis, Lyme disease, "tick fever," Rocky Mountain spotted fever and babesiosis. All are important diseases which need to be prevented whenever possible.

This is only possible by limiting the exposure of our pets to ticks.

For those species of tick that dwell indoors, the eggs are laid mostly in cracks and on vertical surfaces in kennels and homes. Otherwise most other species are found outside in vegetation, such as grassy meadows, woods, brush, and weeds.

Ticks feed only on blood but they don't actually bite. They attach to an animal by sticking their harpoon-shaped mouthparts into the animal's skin and then they suck blood. Some ticks can increase their size 20-50 times as they feed. Favorite places for them to locate are between the toes and in the ears although they can appear anywhere on the skin surface.

A good approach to prevent ticks is to remove underbrush and leaf litter, and to thin the trees in areas where dogs are allowed. This removes the cover and food sources for small mammals that serve as hosts for ticks. Ticks must have adequate cover that provides high levels of moisture and at the same time provides an opportunity of contact with animals. Keeping the lawn well maintained also makes ticks less likely to drop by and stay.

Because of the potential for ticks to transmit a variety of harmful diseases, dogs should be carefully inspected after walks through wooded areas (where ticks may be found) and careful removal of all ticks can be very important in the prevention of disease. Care should be taken not to squeeze, crush, or puncture the body of the tick since exposure to body fluids of ticks may lead to spread of any disease carried by that tick to the animal or to the person removing the tick. The tick should be disposed of in a container of alcohol or flushed down the toilet. If the site becomes infected, veterinary attention should be sought immediately. Insecticides and repellents should only be applied to pets following appropriate veterinary advice, since indiscriminate use can be dangerous. Recently, a new tick collar has become available which contains amitraz. This collar not only kills ticks, but causes them to retract from the skin within two to three days. This greatly reduces the chances of ticks transmitting a variety of diseases. A spray formulation has also recently been developed and marketed. It might seem that there should be vaccines for all the diseases carried by ticks but only a Lyme disease (*Borrelia burgdorferi*) formulation is currently available.

MANGE

Mange refers to any skin condition caused by mites. The contagious mites include ear mites, scabies mites, *Cheyletiella* mites and chiggers. Demodectic mange is associated with proliferation of *Demodex* mites, but they are not considered contagious.

The most common causes of mange in dogs are ear mites and these are extremely contagious. The best way to avoid ear mites is to buy pups from sources that don't have a problem with ear mite infestation. Otherwise, pups readily acquire them when kept in crowded environments in which other animals might be carriers. Treatment is effective if whole body (or systemic) therapy is used, but relapses are common when medication in the ear canal is the only approach. This is because the mites tend to crawl out of the ear canal when medications are instilled. They simply feed elsewhere on the body until it is safe for them to return to the ears.

Scabies mites and *Cheyletiella* mites are passed on by other dogs that are carrying the mites. They are "social" diseases that can be prevented by preventing exposure of your dog to others that are infested. Scabies (sarcoptic mange) has the dubi-

ous honor of being the most itchy disease to which dogs are susceptible. Chigger mites are present in forested areas and dogs acquire them by roaming in these areas. All can be effectively diagnosed and treated by your veterinarian should your dog happen to become infested.

HEARTWORM

Heartworm disease is caused by the worm *Dirofilaria immitis* and is spread by mosquitoes. The female heartworms produce microfilariae (baby worms) that circulate in the bloodstream, waiting to by picked up by mosquitoes to pass the infection along. Dogs do not get heartworm by socializing with infected dogs; they only get infected by mosquitoes that carry the infective microfilariae. The adult heartworms grow in the heart and major blood vessels and eventually cause heart failure.

Fortunately, heartworm is easily prevented by safe oral medications that can be administered daily or on a once-a-month basis. The once-a-month preparations also help prevent many of the common intestinal parasites, such as hookworms, roundworms and whipworms.

Prior to giving any preventative medication for heartworm, an antigen test (an immunologic test that detects heartworms) should be performed by a veterinarian since it is dangerous to give the medication to dogs that harbor the parasite. Some experts also recommend a microfilarial test, just to be doubly certain. Once the test results show that the dog is free of heartworms, the preventative therapy can be commenced. The length of time the heartworm preventatives must be given depends on the length of the mosquito season. In some parts of the country, dogs are on preventative therapy year round. Heartworm vaccines may soon be available but the preventatives now available are easy to administer, inexpensive and quite safe.

Roundworms are spaghetti-like worms that cause a potbellied appearance and a dull coat, along with more severe symptoms, such as diarrhea and vomiting. Photo courtesy of Merck Ag Vet.

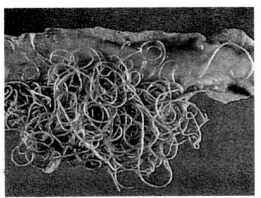

INTESTINAL PARASITES

The most important internal parasites in dogs are roundworms, hookworms, tapeworms and whipworms. Roundworms are the most common. It has been estimated that 13 trillion roundworm eggs are discharged in dog feces every day! Studies have shown that 75% of all pups carry roundworms and start shedding them by three weeks of age. People are infected by exposure to dog feces containing infective roundworm eggs, not by handling pups. Hookworms can cause a disorder known as *cutaneous larva migrans* in people. In dogs, they are most dangerous to puppies since they latch onto the intestines and suck blood. They can cause anemia and even death when they are present in large numbers. The most common tapeworm is *Dipylidium caninum* which is spread by fleas. However, another tapeworm (*Echinococcus multilocularis*) can cause fatal disease in people and can be spread to people from dogs. Whipworms live in the lower aspects of the intestines. Dogs get whipworms by consuming infective larvae. However, it may be another three months before they start shedding them in their stool, greatly complicating diagnosis. In other words, dogs can be infected by whipworms, but fecal evaluations are usually negative until the dog starts passing those eggs three months after being infected.

Other parasites, such as coccidia, *Cryptosporidium*, *Giardia* and flukes can also cause problems in dogs. The best way to prevent all internal parasite problems is to have pups dewormed according to your veterinarian's recommendations, and to have parasite checks done on a regular basis, at least annually.

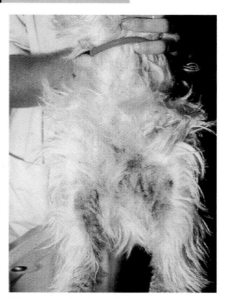

Skin conditions like mange can leave a dog's coat infected, itchy and raw. Mange can be effectively diagnosed and treated by your veterinarian.

VIRAL INFECTIONS

Dogs get viral infections such as distemper, hepatitis, parvovirus and rabies by exposure to infected animals. The key to prevention is controlled exposure to other animals and, of course, vaccination. Today's vaccines are extremely effective and properly vaccinated dogs are at minimal risk for contracting these diseases. However, it is still important to limit exposure to other animals that might be harboring infection. When selecting a facility for boarding or grooming an animal, make sure they limit their clientele to animals that have documented vaccine histories. This is in everyone's best interest. Similarly, make sure your veterinarian has a quarantine area for infected dogs and that animals aren't admitted for surgery, boarding, grooming or diagnostic testing without up-to-date vaccinations. By controlling exposure and ensuring vaccination, your pet should be safe from these potentially devastating diseases.

It is beyond the scope of this book to settle all the controversies of vaccination but they are

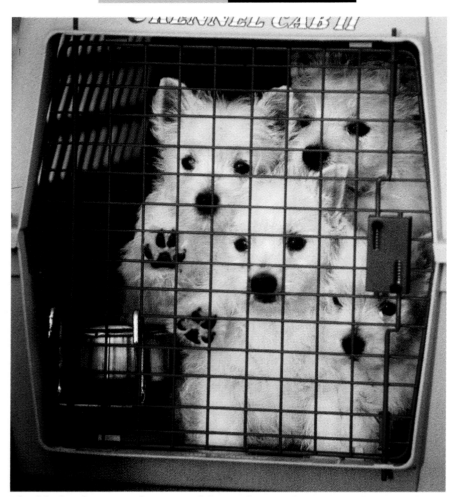

Viral infections can be passed from dog to dog, so make sure dogs that board or live together in close quarters have received the proper vaccinations.

worth mentioning. Should vaccines be combined in a single injection? It's convenient and cheaper to do it this way, but might some vaccine ingredients interfere with others? Some say yes, some say no. Are vaccine schedules designed for convenience or effectiveness? Mostly convenience. Some ingredients may only need to be given every two or more years. Research is incomplete. Should the dose of the vaccine vary with weight or should a West Highland White Terrier receive the same dose as a Great Dane? Good questions, no definitive answers. Finally, should we be using modified-live or inactivated vaccine products? There is no short answer for this debate. Ask your veterinarian and do a lot of reading yourself!

CANINE COUGH

Canine infectious tracheobronchitis, also known as canine cough and kennel cough, is a contagious viral/bacterial disease that results in a hacking cough that may persist for many weeks. It is common wherever dogs are kept in close quarters, such as kennels, pet stores, grooming parlors, dog shows, training classes, and even veterinary clinics. The condition doesn't respond well to most medications, but eventually clears spontaneously over a course of many weeks. Pneumonia is a possible but uncommon complication.

Prevention is best achieved by limiting exposure and utilizing vaccination. The fewer opportunities you give your dog to contact others, the less the likelihood of getting infected. Vaccination is not foolproof because many different viruses can be involved. Parainfluenza virus is

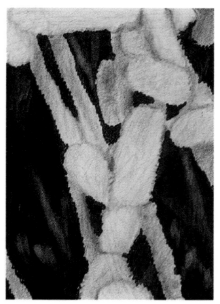

Bordetella attached to canine cilia. Otherwise known as kennel cough, this disease is highly contagious and should be vaccinated against routinely.

included in most vaccines and is one of the more common viruses known to initiate the condition. *Bordetella bronchiseptica* is the bacterium most often associated with tracheobronchitis and a vaccine is now available that needs to be repeated twice yearly for dogs at risk. This vaccine is squirted into the nostrils to help stop the infection before it gets deeper into the respiratory tract. Make sure the vaccination is given several days (preferably two weeks) before exposure to ensure maximal protection.

FIRST AID

by Judy Iby, RVT

**KNOWING YOUR DOG
IN GOOD HEALTH**

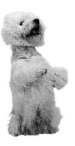

With some experience, you will learn how to give your dog a physical at home, and consequently will learn to recognize many potential problems. If you can detect a problem early, you can seek timely medical help and thereby decrease your dog's risk of developing a more serious problem.

Facing page: Puppies are very vunerable to outside dangers! Always keep a close eye on your West Highland White Terrier.

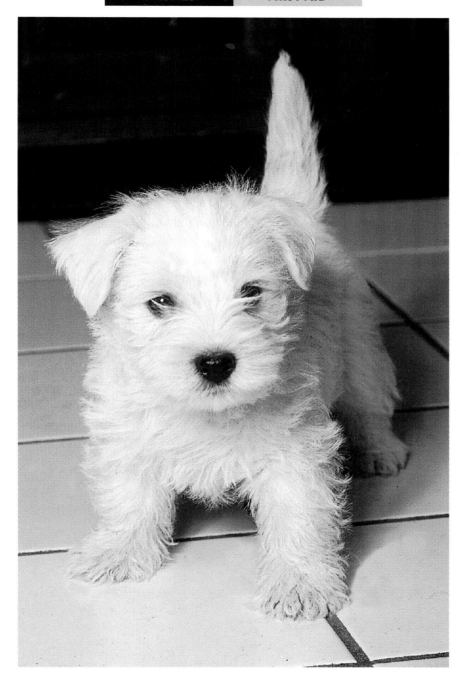

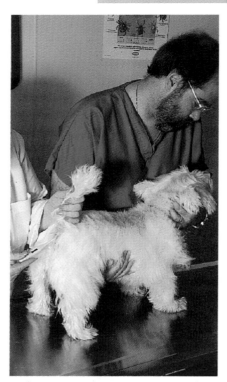

It is easy to take your Westie's temperature in the standing position. A dog's normal temperature is between 100.5 and 102.5 degrees Fahrenheit.

Every pet owner should be able to take his pet's temperature, pulse, respirations, and check the capillary refill time (CRT). Knowing what is normal will alert the pet owner to what is abnormal, and this can be life saving for the sick pet.

TEMPERATURE

The dog's normal temperature is 100.5 to 102.5 degrees Fahrenheit. Take the temperature rectally for at least one minute. Be sure to shake the thermometer down first, and you may find it helpful to lubricate the end. It is easy to take the temperature with the dog in a standing position. Be sure to hold on to the thermometer so that it isn't expelled or sucked in. A dog could have an elevated temperature if he is excited or if he is overheated; however, a high temperature could indicate a medical emergency. On the other hand, if the temperature is below 100 degrees, this could also indicate an emergency.

CAPILLARY REFILL TIME AND GUM COLOR

It is important to know how your dog's gums look when he is healthy, so you will be able to recognize a difference if he is not feeling well. There are a few breeds, among them the Chow Chow and its relatives, that have black gums and a black tongue. This is normal for them. In general, a healthy dog will have bright pink gums. Pale gums are an indication of shock or anemia and are an emergency. Likewise, any yellowish tint is an indication of a sick dog. To check capillary refill time (CRT) press your thumb against the dog's gum. The gum will blanch out (turn white) but should refill (return to the normal pink color) in one to two seconds. CRT is very important. If the refill time is slow and your dog is acting poorly, you should call your veterinarian immediately.

HEART RATE, PULSE, AND RESPIRATIONS

Heart rate depends on the breed of the dog and his health. Normal heart rates range from about 50 beats per minute in the larger breeds to 130 beats per minute in the smaller breeds. You can take the heart rate by pressing your fingertips on the dog's chest. Count for either 10 or 15 seconds, and then multiply by either 6 or 4 to obtain the rate per minute. A normal pulse is the same as the heart rate and is taken at the femoral artery located on the insides of both rear legs. Respirations should be observed and depending on the size and breed of the dog should be 10 to 30 per minute. Obviously, illness or excitement could account for abnormal rates.

PREPARING FOR AN EMERGENCY

It is a good idea to prepare for an emergency by making a list and keeping it by the phone. This list should include:
1. Your veterinarian's name,

address, phone number, and office hours.
2. Your veterinarian's policy for after-hour care. Does he take his own emergencies or does he refer them to an emergency clinic?
3. The name, address, phone number and hours of the emergency clinic your veterinarian uses.
4. The number of the National Poison Control Center for Animals in Illinois: 1-800-

A healthy Westie should have pink, firm gums. Pale gums are an indication of shock or anemia and should be considered an emergency.

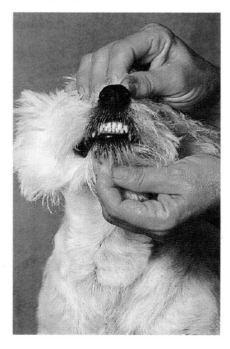

548-2423. It is open 24 hours a day.

In a true emergency, time is of the essence. Some signs of an emergency may be:

1. Pale gums or an abnormal heart rate.
2. Abnormal temperature, lower than 100 degrees or over 104 degrees.
3. Shock or lethargy.
4. Spinal paralysis.

A dog hit by a car needs to be checked out and probably should have radiographs of the chest and abdomen to rule out pneumothorax or ruptured bladder.

EMERGENCY MUZZLE

An injured, frightened dog may not even recognize his owner and may be inclined to bite. If your dog should be injured, you may need to muzzle him to protect yourself before you try to handle him. It is a good idea to practice muzzling the calm, healthy dog so you understand the technique. Slip a lead over his head for control. You can tie his mouth shut with something like a two-foot-long bandage or piece of cloth. A necktie, stocking, leash or even a piece of rope will also work.

1. Make a large loop by tying a loose knot in the middle of the bandage or cloth.
2. Hold the ends up, one in each hand.
3. Slip the loop over the dog's muzzle and lower jaw, just behind his nose.
4. Quickly tighten the loop so he can't open his mouth.
5. Tie the ends under his lower jaw.
6. Make a knot there and pull the ends back on each side of his face, under the ears, to the back of his head.

If he should start to vomit, you will need to remove the muzzle immediately. Otherwise, he could aspirate vomitus into his lungs.

ANTIFREEZE POISONING

Antifreeze in the driveway is a potential killer. Because antifreeze is sweet, dogs will lap it up. The active ingredient in antifreeze is ethylene glycol, which causes irreversible kidney damage. If you witness your pet ingesting antifreeze, you should call your veterinarian immediately. He may recommend that you induce vomiting at once by using hydrogen peroxide, or he may recommend a test to confirm antifreeze ingestion. Treatment is aggressive and must be administered promptly if the dog is to live, but you wouldn't want to subject your dog to unnecessary treatment.

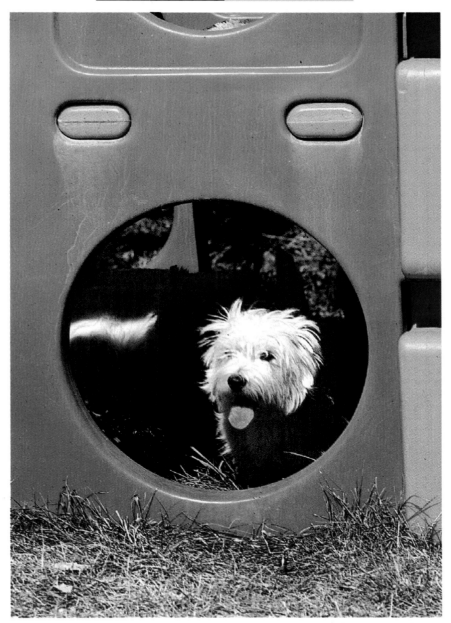

These two Westies are able to get away from the sun while enjoying the playground, so they can stay cool.

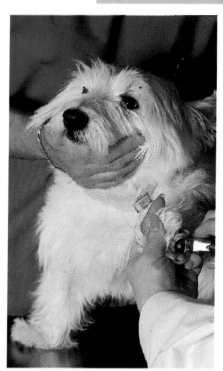

When trimming your dogs nails, be careful not to cut the "quick." If bleeding does occur, styptic powder can be used to control it.

BEE STINGS

A severe reaction to a bee sting (anaphylaxis) can result in difficulty breathing, collapse and even death. A symptom of a bee sting is swelling around the muzzle and face. Bee stings are antihistamine responsive. Over-the-counter antihistamines are available Ask your veterinarian for recommendations on safe antihistamines to use and doses to administer. You should moni-

tor the dog's gum color and respirations and watch for a decrease in swelling. If your dog is showing signs of anaphylaxis, your veterinarian may need to give him an injection of corticosteroids. It would be wise to call your veterinarian and confirm treatment.

BLEEDING

Bleeding can occur in many forms, such as a ripped dewclaw, a toenail cut too short, a puncture wound, a severe laceration, etc. If a pressure bandage is needed, it must be released every 15-20 minutes. Be careful of elastic bandages since it is easy to apply them too tightly. Any bandage material should be clean. If no regular bandage is available, a small towel or wash cloth can be used to cover the wound and bind it with a necktie, scarf, or something similar. Styptic powder, or even a soft cake of soap, can be used to stop a bleeding toenail. A ripped dewclaw or toenail may need to be cut back by the veterinarian and possibly treated with antibiotics. Depending on their severity, lacerations and puncture wounds may also need professional treatment. Your first thought should be to clean the wound with peroxide, soap and water, or some other antiseptic cleanser. Don't use alcohol since it deters the healing of the tissue.

BLOAT

Although not generally considered a first aid situation, bloat can occur in a dog rather suddenly. Truly, it is an emergency! Gastric dilatation-volvulus or gastric torsion—the twisting of the stomach to cut off both entry and exit, causing the organ to "bloat," is a disorder primarily found in the larger, more deep-chested breeds. It is life threatening and requires immediate veterinary assistance.

BURNS

If your dog gets a chemical burn, call your veterinarian immediately. Rinse any other burns with cold water and if the burn is significant, call your veterinarian. It may be necessary to clip the hair around the burn so it will be easier to keep clean. You can cleanse the wound on a daily basis with saline and apply a topical antimicrobial ointment, such as silver sulfadiazine 1 percent cream or gentamicin cream. Burns can be debilitating, especially to an older pet. They can cause pain and shock. It takes about three weeks for the skin to slough after the burn and there is the possibility of permanent hair loss.

CARDIOPULMONARY RESUSCITATION (CPR)

Check to see if your dog has a heart beat, pulse and spontaneous respiration. If his pupils are already dilated and fixed, the prognosis is less favorable. This is an emergency situation that requires two people to administer lifesaving techniques. One person needs to breathe for the dog while the other person tries to establish heart rhythm. Mouth to mouth resuscitation starts with two initial breaths, one to one and a half seconds in duration. After the initial breaths, breathe for the dog once after every five chest compressions. (You do not want to expand the dog's lungs while his chest is being compressed.) You inhale, cover the dog's nose with your mouth, and exhale *gently*. You should see the dog's chest expand. Sometimes, pulling the tongue forward stimulates respiration. You should be ventilating the dog 12-20 times per minute. The person managing the chest compressions should have the dog lying on his right side with one hand on either side of the dog's chest, directed over the heart between the fourth and fifth ribs (usually this is the point of the flexed elbow). The number of compressions administered depends on the size

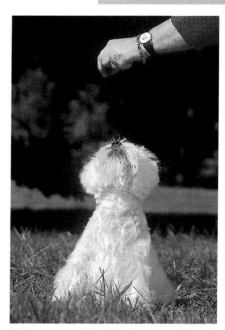

Allow your Westie the occasional treat, but do not give him human food, especially chocolate. Chocolate can be toxic to your pet.

mine, overstimulate the dog's nervous system. Ten ounces of milk chocolate can kill a 12-pound dog. Symptoms of poisoning include restlessness, vomiting, increased heart rate, seizure, and coma. Death is possible. If your dog has ingested chocolate, you can give syrup of ipecac at a dosage of one-eighth of a teaspoon per pound to induce vomiting. Two tablespoons of hydrogen peroxide is an alternative treatment.

CHOKING

You need to open the dog's mouth to see if any object is visible. Try to hold him upside down to see if the object can be dislodged. While you are working on your dog, call your veterinarian, as time may be critical.

of the patient. Attempt 80-120 compressions per minute. Check for spontaneous respiration and/ or heart beat. If present, monitor the patient and discontinue resuscitation. If you haven't already done so, call your veterinarian at once and make arrangements to take your pet in for professional treatment.

DOG BITES

If your dog is bitten, wash the area and determine the severity of the situation. Some bites may need immediate attention, for instance, if it is bleeding profusely or if a lung is punctured. Other bites may be only superficial scrapes. Most dog bite cases need to be seen by the veterinarian, and some may require antibiotics. It is important that you learn if the offending dog has had a rabies vaccination. This is important for your dog, but also

CHOCOLATE TOXICOSIS

Dogs like chocolate, but chocolate kills dogs. Its two basic chemicals, caffeine and theobro-

for you, in case you are the victim. Wash the wound and call your doctor for further instructions. You should check on your tetanus vaccination history. Rarely, and I mean rarely, do dogs get tetanus. If the offending dog is a stray, try to confine him for observation. He will need

DROWNING

Remove any debris from the dog's mouth and swing the dog, holding him upside down. Stimulate respiration by pulling his tongue forward. Administer CPR if necessary, and call your veterinarian. Don't give up working on the dog. Be sure to wrap

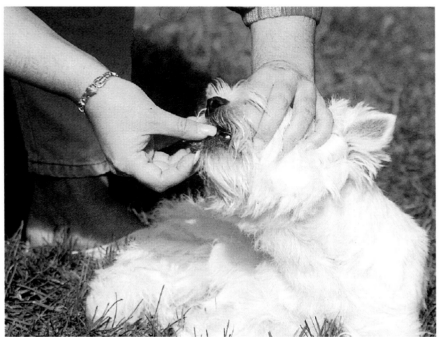

In order to prevent choking, remove all foreign objects from your dog's mouth.

to be confined for ten days. A dog that has bitten a human and is not current on his rabies vaccination cannot receive a rabies vaccination for ten days. Dog bites should be reported to the Board of Health.

him in blankets if he is cold or in shock.

ELECTROCUTION

You may want to look into puppy proofing your house by installing GFCIs (Ground Fault

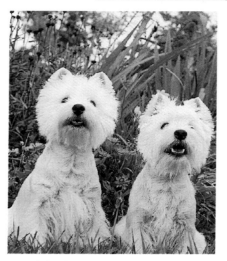

Familiarize yourself with the plants found in your yard. Some plants are poisonous to your Westie, so never leave him outside unsupervised.

Circuit Interrupters) on your electrical outlets. A GFCI just saved my dog's life. He had pulled an extension cord into his crate and was "teething" on it at seven years of age. The GFCI kept him from being electrocuted. Turn off the current before touching the dog. Resuscitate him by administering CPR and pulling his tongue forward to stimulate respiration. Try mouth-to-mouth breathing if the dog is not breathing. Take him to your veterinarian as soon as possible since electrocution can cause internal problems, such as lung damage, which need medical treatment.

EYES

Red eyes indicate inflammation, and any redness to the upper white part of the eye (sclera) may constitute an emergency. Squinting, cloudiness to the cornea, or loss of vision could indicate severe problems, such as glaucoma, anterior uveitis and episcleritis. Glaucoma is an emergency if you want to save the dog's eye. A prolapsed third eyelid is abnormal and is a symptom of an underlying problem. If something should get in your dog's eye, flush it out with cold water or a saline eye wash. Epiphora and allergic conjunctivitis are annoying and frequently persistent problems. Epiphora (excessive tearing) leaves the area below the eye wet and sometimes stained. The wetness may lead to a bacterial infection. There are numerous causes (allergies, infections, foreign matter, abnormally located eyelashes and adjacent facial hair that rubs against the eyeball, defects or diseases of the tear drainage system, birth defects of the eyelids, etc.) and the treatment is based on the cause. Keeping the hair around the eye cut short and sponging the eye daily will give relief. Many cases are responsive to medical treatment. Allergic conjunctivitis may be a seasonal problem if the dog has inhalant allergies (e.g., ragweed), or it may be a year 'round problem. The conjunctiva becomes red and swollen and is prone to a bacterial infection associated with mucus accumulation or pus in the eye. Again keeping the hair around the eyes short will give relief. Mild corticosteroid drops or ointment will also give relief. The underlying problem should be investigated.

FISH HOOKS

An imbedded fish hook will probably need to be removed by the veterinarian. More than likely, sedation will be required along with antibiotics. Don't try to remove it yourself. The shank of the hook will need to be cut off

in order to push the other end through.

FOREIGN OBJECTS

I can't tell you how many chicken bones my first dog ingested. Fortunately she had a "cast iron stomach" and never suffered the consequences. However, she was always going to the veterinarian for treatment. Not all dogs are so lucky. It is unbelievable what some dogs will take a liking to. I have assisted in surgeries in which all kinds of foreign objects were removed from the stomach and/or intestinal tract. Those objects included socks, pantyhose, stockings, clothing, diapers, sanitary products, plastic, toys, and, last

A Roar-Hide® chew is great for your Westie to munch on. Not only is it completely edible, but it will not break into small pieces that your dog might choke on.

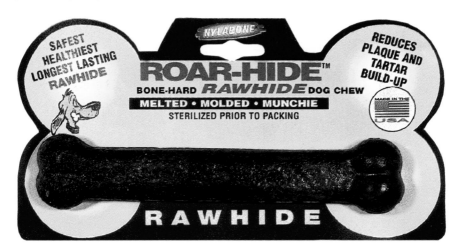

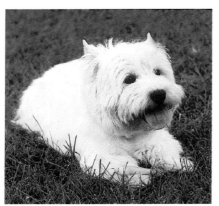

Give your dog a Nylabone® to play with. The Petite size is perfect for your adorable Westie.

but not least, rawhides. Surgery is costly and not always successful, especially if it is performed too late. If you see or suspect your dog has ingested a foreign object, contact your veterinarian immediately. He may tell you to induce vomiting or he may have you bring your dog to the clinic immediately. Don't induce vomiting without the veterinarian's permission, since the object may cause more damage on the way back up than it would if you allow it to pass through.

HEATSTROKE

Heatstroke is an emergency! The classic signs are rapid, shallow breathing; rapid heartbeat; a temperature above 104 degrees; and subsequent collapse. The dog needs to be cooled as quickly as possible and treated immediately by the veterinarian. If possible, spray him down with cool water and pack ice around his head, neck, and groin. Monitor his temperature and stop the cooling process as soon as his temperature reaches 103 degrees. Nevertheless, you will need to keep monitoring his temperature to be sure it doesn't elevate again. If the temperature continues to drop to below 100 degrees, it could be life threatening. Get professional help immediately. Prevention is more successful than treatment. Those at the greatest risk are brachycephalic (short nosed) breeds, obese dogs, and those that suffer from cardiovascular disease. Dogs are not able to cool off by sweating as people can. Their only way is through panting and radiation of heat from the skin surface. When stressed and exposed to high environmental temperature, high humidity, and poor ventilation, a dog can suffer heatstroke very quickly. Many people do not realize how quickly a car can overheat. Never leave a dog unattended in a car. It is even against the law in some states. Also, a brachycephalic, obese, or infirm dog should never be left unattended outside during inclement weather and should have his activities curtailed. Any dog left outside, by law, must be assured adequate shelter (including shade) and fresh water.

POISONS

Try to locate the source of the poison (the container which lists the ingredients) and call your veterinarian immediately. Be prepared to give the age and weight of your dog, the quantity of poison consumed and the probable time of ingestion. Your veterinarian will want you to read off the ingredients. If you can't reach him, you can call a local poison center or the National Poison Control Center for Animals in Illinois, which is open 24 hours a day. Their phone number is 1-800-548-2423. There is a charge for their service, so you may need to have a credit card number available.

Symptoms of poisoning include muscle trembling and weakness, increased salivation, vomiting and loss of bowel control. There are numerous household toxins (over 500,000). A dog can be poisoned by toxins in the garbage. Other poisons include pesticides, pain relievers, prescription drugs, plants, chocolate, and cleansers. Since I own small dogs I don't have to worry about my dogs jumping up to the kitchen counters, but when I owned a large breed she would clean the counter, eating all the prescription medications.

Your pet can be poisoned by means other than directly ingesting the toxin. Ingesting a rodent that has ingested a rodenticide is one example. It is possible for a dog to have a reaction to the pesticides used by exterminators. If this is suspected you should contact the exterminator about the potential dangers of the pesticides used and their side effects.

Don't give human drugs to your dog unless your veterinarian has given his approval. Some human medications can be deadly to dogs.

Make sure your dogs have plenty of cool water and shade when outside to prevent heatstroke.

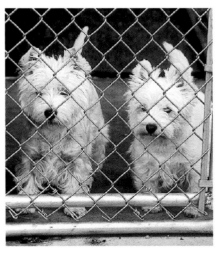

POISONOUS PLANTS

Amaryllis (bulb)	Jasmine (berries)
Andromeda	Jerusalem Cherry
Apple Seeds (cyanide)	Jimson Weed
Arrowgrass	Laburnum
Avocado	Larkspur
Azalea	Laurel
Bittersweet	Locoweed
Boxwood	Marigold
Buttercup	Marijuana
Caladium	Mistletoe (berries)
Castor Bean	Monkshood
Cherry Pits	Mushrooms
Chokecherry	Narcissus (bulb)
Climbing Lily	Nightshade
Crown of Thorns	Oleander
Daffodil (bulb)	Peach
Daphne	Philodendron
Delphinium	Poison Ivy
Dieffenbachia	Privet
Dumb Cane	Rhododendron
Elephant Ear	Rhubarb
English Ivy	Snow on
Elderberry	the Mountain
Foxglove	Stinging Nettle
Hemlock	Toadstool
Holly	Tobacco
Hyacinth (bulb)	Tulip (bulb)
Hydrangea	Walnut
Iris (bulb)	Wisteria
Japanese Yew	Yew

This list was published in the American Kennel Club *Gazette*, February, 1995. As the list states these are common poisonous plants, but this list may not be complete. If your dog ingests a poisonous plant, try to identify it and call your veterinarian. Some plants cause more harm than others.

PORCUPINE QUILLS

Removal of quills is best left up to your veterinarian since it can be quite painful. Your unhappy dog would probably appreciate being sedated for the removal of the quills.

SEIZURE (CONVULSION OR FIT)

Many breeds, including mixed breeds, are predisposed to seizures, although a seizure may be secondary to an underlying medical condition. Usually a seizure is not considered an emergency unless it lasts longer than ten minutes. Nevertheless, you should notify your veterinarian. Dogs do not swallow their tongues. Do not handle the dog's mouth since your dog probably cannot control his actions and may inadvertently bite you. The seizure can be mild; for instance, a dog can have a seizure standing up. More frequently the dog will lose consciousness and may urinate and/or defecate. The best thing you can do for your dog is to put him in a safe place or to block off the stairs or areas where he can fall.

SHOCK

Shock is a life threatening condition and requires immediate veterinary care. It can occur after an injury or even after severe fright. Other causes of shock are hemorrhage, fluid loss, sepsis, toxins, adrenal insufficiency, cardiac failure, and anaphylaxis. The symptoms are a rapid weak pulse, shallow breathing, dilated pupils, subnormal temperature, and muscle weakness.

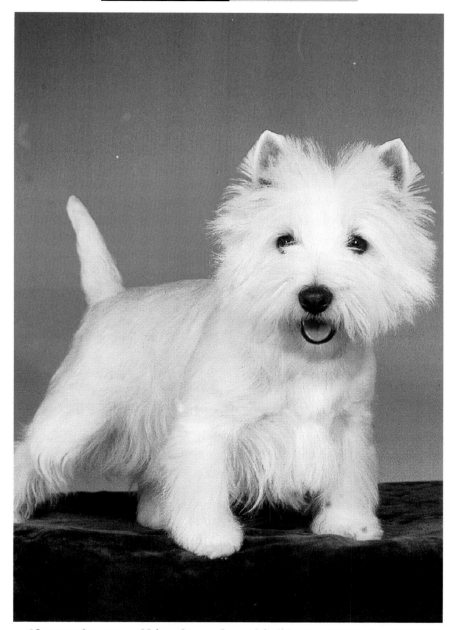

If you take care of him throughout his life, your Westie will be the healthy, spunky dog you hoped he would be.

The capillary refill time (CRT) is slow, taking longer than two seconds for normal gum color to return. Keep the dog warm while transporting him to the veterinary clinic. Time is critical for survival.

SKUNKS

Skunk spraying is not necessarily an emergency, although it would be in my house. If the dog's eyes are sprayed, you need to rinse them well with water. One remedy for deskunking the dog is to wash him in tomato juice and follow with a soap and water bath. The newest remedy is bathing the dog in a mixture of one quart of three percent hydrogen peroxide, quarter cup baking soda, and one teaspoon liquid soap. Rinse well. There are also commercial products available.

SNAKE BITES

It is always a good idea to know what poisonous snakes reside in your area. Rattlesnakes, water moccasins, copperheads, and coral snakes are residents of some areas of the United States. Pack ice around the area that is bitten and call your veterinarian immediately to alert him that you are on your way. Try to identify the snake or at least be able to describe it (for the use of

antivenin). It is possible that he may send you to another clinic that has the proper antivenin.

SEVERE TRAUMA

See that the dog's head and neck are extended so if the dog is unconscious or in shock, he is able to breathe. If there is any vomitus, you should try to get the head extended down with the body elevated to prevent vomitus from being aspirated. Alert your veterinarian that you are on your way.

TOAD POISONING

Bufo toads are quite deadly. You should find out if these nasty little critters are native to your area.

VACCINATION REACTION

Once in a while, a dog may suffer an anaphylactic reaction to a vaccine. Symptoms include swelling around the muzzle, extending to the eyes. Your veterinarian may ask you to return to his office to determine the severity of the reaction. It is possible that your dog may need to stay at the hospital for a few hours during future vaccinations.

RECOMMENDED READING

DR. ACKERMAN'S DOG BOOKS FROM T.F.H.

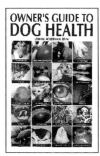

OWNER'S GUIDE TO DOG HEALTH
TS-214, 432 pages
Over 300 color photographs
Winner of the 1995 Dog Writers Association of America's Best Health Book, this comprehensive title gives accurate, up-to-date information on all the major disorders and conditions found in dogs. Completely illustrated to help owners visualize signs of illness, different states of infection, procedures and treatment, it covers nutrition, skin disorders, disorders of the major body systems (reproductive, digestive, respiratory), eye problems, vaccines and vaccinations, dental health and more.

DOG BEHAVIOR AND TRAINING
Veterinary Advice for Owners
TS-252, 292 pages
Over 200 color photographs
Joined by co-editors Gary Landsberg, DVM and Wayne Hunthausen, DVM, Dr. Ackerman and about 20 experts in behavioral studies and training set forth a practical guide to the common problems owners experience with their dogs. Since behavioral disorders are the number-one reason for owners to abandon a dog, it is essential for owners to understand how the dog thinks and how to correct him if he misbehaves. The book cover socialization, selection, rewards and punishment, puppy-problem prevention, excitable and disobedient behaviors, sexual behaviors, aggression, children, stress and more.

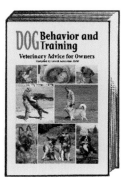

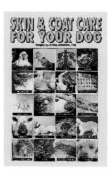

SKIN & COAT CARE FOR YOUR DOG
TS-249 224 pages
Over 200 color photographs
Dr. Ackerman, a specialist in the field of dermatology and a Diplomate of the American College of Veterinary Dermatology, joins 14 of the world's most respected dermatologists and other experts to produce an extremely helpful manual on the dog's skin. Coat and skin problems are extremely common in the dog, and owners need to better understand the conditions that affect their dog's coats. The book details everything from the basics of parasites and mange to grooming techniques, medications, hair loss and more.

RECOMMENDED READING

OTHER DOG BOOKS FROM T.F.H.

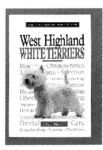

A NEW OWNER'S GUIDE TO WEST HIGHLAND WHITE TERRIERS
by Dawn Martin
JG-116, 160 pages
Over 150 full color photographs
Provides the West Highland White Terrier owner with detailed and concise information from history to puppy care to training and management. Topics covered include selection, feeding and health care.

BOOK OF THE WEST HIGHLAND WHITE TERRIER
by Anna K. Nicholas
TS-187, 224 pages
Over 190 full color photographs
Anna K. Nicholas is one of America's most famous dog show judges and has a long association with the Westie. In The Book of the West Highland White Terrier she offers useful advice on raising, training and grooming. The book remains valuable for its impressive collection of historical photographs and the information about the dogs in them.

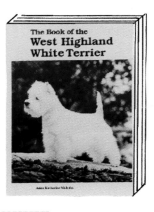

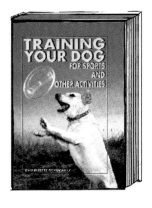

TRAINING YOUR DOG FOR SPORTS AND OTHER ACTIVITIES
by Charlotte Schwartz
TS-258, 160 pages
Over 200 full-color photographs
In this colorful and vividly illustrated book, author Charlotte Schwartz, a professional dog trainer for 40 years, demonstrates how your pet dog can assume a useful and meaningful role in everyday life. No matter what lifestyle you lead or what kind of dog you share your life with, there's a suitable and eyeopening activity in this book for you and your dog.